The Emotional
First Aid Manual

by Janet Buell
Foreword by Frank A. Gerbode, M.D.
Introduction by Robert H. Moore, Ph.D.
Large-Scale Trauma by William C. Foreman, Ph.D.

The Emotional First Aid Manual

by Janet Buell
Foreword by Frank A. Gerbode, M.D.
Introduction by Robert H. Moore, Ph.D.
Large-Scale Trauma by William C. Foreman, Ph.D.

This book is dedicated to all the caregivers in the world
who strive to help their fellow man

Published by Innovations Press
1st Edition

Copyright 2006 by Janet Buell

Library of Congress Cataloging-in-Publication Data

Buell, Janet, 1945-
The emotional first aid manual / by Janet Buell ; foreword by
Frank Gerbode ; introduction by Robert Moore ; Large-scale trauma,
by Clay Foreman. -- 1st ed.
    p. cm.
Includes bibliographical references and index.
ISBN-13: 978-1-929830-15-2 (alk. paper)
ISBN-10: 1-929830-15-7 (alk. paper)
1. Crisis intervention (Mental health services) I. Title.
  RC480.6.B84 2006
  362.2'04251--dc22

                                    2006023200

ISBN 1-929830-15-7
ISBN 978-1-929830-15-2

Table of Contents

Foreword

By Robert H. Moore, PhD

Can a lay person render emotional first aid as effectively as a professional counselor?

Without a doubt!

Just as it doesn't take a physician to dress a wound or a dentist to clean your teeth, it doesn't take a social worker or psychologist to respond effectively to someone in an emotional crisis. All it takes is a clear head, a caring heart and a little training. In fact, it may surprise you how uncomplicated it often is to help someone in emotional distress feel a whole lot better.

One can learn a great deal about the basics of rendering help of this sort from a good, volunteer crisis counselor's workshop, sometimes in just a few weeks. The best such workshops give participants plenty of opportunity to hone their new skills with each other over the course of the program. Many turn out volunteer counselors whose emotional first aid is fully as effective as that of their professional counterparts.

How can that be?

Consider what it takes to become a professional counselor. The curriculum of the average, two-year, masters level, counseling or social service program is not devoted entirely to developing its students' counseling skills. Graduate degree programs in the helping professions include a wide variety of theoretical, historic and regulatory subjects. These meet the requirements of state professional boards and prepare students for their licensing examinations. Graduate programs also provide their students with opportunities to practice their new skills. These are called "internships" or "practica". But graduate students at both the masters and doctoral levels know from the start that the day they receive their diplomas, their clinical training will just have begun. In this regard, they are very much like recent medical school graduates. They have their degrees and licenses in hand, but their most valuable clinical skills remain to be developed.

In any case, it's not at all uncommon for a good crisis counselor's workshop, unburdened by courses that: a) trace human psychosocial development from birth to old age, b) define and differentiate the principal psychodiagnostic categories, and c) survey the philosophic contributions of every major behavioral theorist from Freud to Ellis — to take its trainees from ground zero to basic counseling proficiency in just a few weeks. Most of the 24-hour rape, abuse, suicide, and addiction "hotlines" from coast to coast are staffed by volunteer counselors who have completed just such programs. The training program for crisis hotline counselors in my area (Pinellas County, Florida), for instance, runs 60 hours. And it's free to those who volunteer.

As for the actual effectiveness of licensed professional versus unlicensed paraprofessional counselors — you should know that studies comparing the counseling proficiencies of graduate mental health workers with those of their lay counterparts have consistently failed to find significant differences between them. Of course, the simple fact that degreed and non-degreed counselors have equally effective basic skills does not mean that formal degree programs really don't count. It means that good training, regardless of where you get it, really does count.

In spite of all this, you should be aware that some licensed professional counselors have what you might call an "attitude" about unlicensed counselors. But don't let that keep you from learning everything you possibly can about emotional first aid, or from freely applying it either! Most of my vigilant professional colleagues are motivated only by a sincere desire to protect the service-seeking consumer from the incompetence of the inadequately trained. So unless you plan to set up a practice, hang out your shingle, represent yourself to the public as a psychotherapist and charge fees for your services (in which case you would need to be licensed), their critical gaze will never linger long in your direction.

Rest assured, you have every right and good reason to learn every-thing there is to know about how best to assist those you love and care for, your friends, neighbors, co-workers, even passers-by in the often difficult business of coping with adversity. As a profes-sional counselor, I would no more take offense at your caring use of "Active Listening", "Values Clarification", or the helpful techniques of NLP or REBT than a physician would resent your timely and ap-propriate use of CPR or the Heimlich maneuver. In fact, if you'll

---

Emotional First Aid Procedures that can be done by Lay People

Active Listening—a term coined by Thomas Gordon, author of the popular *Effectiveness Training* series, to represent the re-flective listening process of Carl Rogers; the basic non-directive or Rogerian approach to counseling.

Values Clarification—an approach to counseling introduced by Sidney Simon, Leland Howe, and Howard Kirschenbaum in their classic book by the same name.

NLP—Neuro-Linguistic Programming: a collection of counter-conditioning strategies first articulated by Richard Bandler and John Grinder in their seminal work, *Frogs into Princes*.

REBT—Rational-Emotive Behavior Therapy (formerly RET); the most popular of the several cognitive-behavior therapies devel-oped by Albert Ellis, author of the perennially popular volume *The New Guide to Rational Living* and several dozen other works.

---

round up a group of your friends and make some sandwiches, I'll come over Saturday and give you a top notch introduction to these subjects myself! Am I serious? Wouldn't your dentist be delighted to hear that you'd brought together a whole room full of people who actually wanted to learn how to floss?

One thing more: you have in hand a most extraordinary volume (for which, in all honesty, I can take absolutely no credit). It contains a compilation of the most useful tips and techniques for handling a wider variety of stressful human circumstances than have ever before been put into print. It's the Bible of emotional first aid — all meat and utterly indispensable to anyone who cares a whit about the well-being of others.

Dr. Robert H. Moore is a 30+ year, licensed mental health counselor, marriage and family therapist and school psychologist. He is board certified in psychotraumatology and crisis intervention. A former, 17-year Director of the Florida branch of the Institute for Rational-Emotive Therapy, he currently confines his practice to corporate crisis consulting.

Introduction

by Frank A. Gerbode, M.D.

Is there a need for "lay" emergency help? Is such help feasible?

The need is certainly obvious. Life is full of trauma and stress for virtually everybody. There is no one I know who has not had some kind of major trauma in his or her life. Most of us have had severe injuries or painful illnesses and operations. We have also experienced the loss—through death, divorce, or disaffection—of someone close to us, and have had other severe personal losses as well. Other incidents continually occur that remind us of previous incidents of loss or pain and force us to painfully relive them. These "reminder" incidents become "secondary traumas" and they add greatly to the burden of life. Most people, then, feel almost continually the effects of their past traumas, and much of human unhappiness is attributable to such unresolved past losses.

Stress and loss is more easily resolved if a person can confront it sooner rather than later. The effect of time is to assist in the process of repression that makes such traumas hard to access and to multiply the aftereffects of such traumas. Time does not heal all wounds. It only covers them up and makes them hard to find, but they continue to fester below the surface. Dealing with such traumas and stresses early on greatly improves the chances that a person will be able to confront and permanently resolve such incidents and renders a more lengthy later handling unnecessary, or at least much easier.

When you address a trauma soon after it has happened, it does not take great expertise to find it and reduce its impact. It has not yet been fully repressed and so is more available than it will ever be again. Thus a very simple procedure can suffice to resolve it at this stage (such as the Compassion Remedy found in this book). Such a procedure is so simple, it is easy to teach it to anyone who wants to help.

When such a primary trauma has been reduced or resolved by means of such "emotional first aid", secondary traumas do not build up on top of it, and the source of a great deal of distress is thus eliminated.

Types of Trauma
Primary Trauma An incident containing pain and/or loss such as an accident, illness, operation, death or abandonment. **Secondary Trauma** An incident that reminds us of earlier incidents containing pain and/or loss.

In that respect, emotional first aid is similar to the physical kind: what you can do at the scene of an accident may be simple, yet lifesaving. It may also prevent permanent disablement or disfigurement and make subsequent treatment much simpler or even unnecessary. A Heimlich maneuver can be lifesaving to a person choking on a piece of food. Otherwise, the person will suffer oxygen deprivation and possible permanent brain damage or death. Likewise, rapid immobilization may prevent further traumatization in the case of a severely broken bone, antidotes or emetics may greatly reduce the trauma from poisoning.

It takes far less skill to use such first-aid procedures than it does to handle the complications that can occur if you don't use them.

And what friends say to friends after a severe trauma can be helpful or harmful. A little training on listening and other skills can make a big difference. You can be even more helpful to your friends if you have some simple yet effective techniques to use to help them than if you mean well but don't know what you are doing. It shouldn't take more than a few hours to teach such techniques to anyone of good will and reasonable intelligence.

Not letting people help other people in a simple way because they might cause harm would be like prohibiting them from rendering first aid: it would actually lead to more harm. People naturally want to help others and they should not, and cannot, be prevented from talking to friends or loved ones who are in distress. A little simple training would tend to reduce the possibility of secondary traumatization from such conversations and increase the beneficial effect of efforts to help that are going to take place anyway.

Will you find this book useful?

Let me ask you the following questions:

A friend has lost her husband in a traffic accident and she's in shock or preoccupied about it. What do you do?

Do you. . .

- try to get her to think about other things, to put her attention on other things in life?

- invite her to delve into why she is so upset about the incident?

- act sympathetic to her and try to be extra nice to her?

- draw her attention to all the positive things she still has going for herself in life?

- give her advice on how to cope with the tragedy?

- tell her all about a similar loss you once had and how you got over it?

- tell her not to be a crybaby?

These are all things that people commonly do in an effort to help. Yet some of these actions are less helpful than others, and some may actually be harmful. If you knew exactly what to do when confronted by a loved one or friend in distress, wouldn't that be a great help to you? Read on and you'll soon know exactly how to render effective and compassionate help!

Frank A. Gerbode, M.D. is a psychiatrist. He is the founder of the Traumatic Incident Reduction Association and author of the book Beyond Psychology — An Introduction to Metapsychology.

Vital Information

There are three primary categories of need for emotional first aid:

1. An immediate loss or trauma that has happened to a person with no history of serious mental illness

2. The acute losses or traumas of the chronically mentally ill

3. Losses and traumas that are compounded by substance abuse (alcohol, drugs, etc.)

Each of the three categories requires a different level of help. It is easiest for the layperson to make a difference in the first category. The immediate trauma and losses of our friends and family are greatly relieved by the "compassionate listening" and "conversational trauma reduction" methods taught in this book.

Often the techniques taught here are all that are needed to bring the friend or loved one to an improved state of emotional health, just as basic first aid can often improve a minor cut or sore to the point where no additional treatment is needed. At other times more help is needed. Each section contains criteria for judging if more aid is required after the initial emotional first-aid procedure is done and a list of resources for obtaining just the right additional aid is contained in the appendix. Section One of this book provides help for those who have suffered an immediate loss or trauma and who have no history of serious mental illness or substance abuse.

For the people who fall into Category Two, the chronically mentally ill, the primary care must naturally be in the hands of a professional health care worker. For friends and family who have not already found a primary source for that help, professional resources and support groups are listed in the appendix.

Even when a chronic mental illness is involved, a layperson can be of some aid in calming the victim and helping to see that he or she receives the professional help they need. Section Two offers useful ways of dealing with acute upsets. These methods have been recommended by support groups and professionals who specialize in each specific illness. Warning signs for those very rare occasions when violence might be a factor are also listed to protect both helper and victim.

People in Category Three, losses and traumas when substance abuse is present, unfortunately are most difficult to help and their care should also be in the hands of a professional health care worker. There are, however, some limited ways in which a layman can help, providing caution is used. Violence and destructive behavior are far more common when drugs or alcohol are involved and the helper must be very aware of his or her own safety. Instructions for the limited care that can be given as well as a listing of resources for professional help are part of Section Three.

Category One:

People who fall in this category are easiest for laypeople to help and will often recover with little or no professional help. Procedures appropriate for Category One are given in Section One and Two of this book.

Category Two:

People who fall in this category can receive limited help from the layperson but need to be under the care of a professional. Procedures appropriate for Category Two are given in Section Three of this book.

Category Three:

People who fall in this category are difficult even for the professional to help and must be handled with great caution. Procedures appropriate for Category Three are given in Section Four of this book.

There are usually two major concerns for the friends and family who seek to provide emotional first aid to their loved ones. The first is that they won't be able to think of anything inspiring or comforting to say. The second is that they might do more harm than good. There is some justification in these concerns. A person trying to perform physical first aid can cause more harm than good if he or she moves a victim with a neck injury, for example. That's why there are a few basic "golden rules" in physical first aid handbooks.

This manual contains some "golden rules" too. The rules that follow are the most important information in this manual. By following these simple rules, you can be certain that you will be able to help—not harm—your loved ones.

Golden Rule #1

Listen—don't talk!

You don't need to say anything inspiring. You only need to know a few simple questions to ask to get the person talking and these questions are provided in the instructions in each section of this book. Then you need to listen to the answers and acknowledge them. In our attempts to help, we all talk too much and listen too little. The ratio of time you spend talking to the time you spend listening should be a maximum of 5% (talking) to 95% (listening). Just recognizing these proportions can take away some of the pressure you might feel to be wise and inspiring.

Golden Rule #2

Be compassionate—not critical

There is nothing helpful in criticizing or judging others. Every bit of good you can do for your fellow human beings will come from your ability to be compassionate. In every loss or trauma are actions or thoughts about which the person may feel guilty or ashamed. Full healing won't occur unless those thoughts can be fully expressed. People who feel they are being judged critically will begin to defend their actions rather than express their thoughts fully. Any time spent defending their actions is wasted time that isn't going to contribute to their healing. It is vital to the person who has been hurt to know that he or she can express any thought, emotion, or deed to the person giving emotional first aid without fear of criticism or judgment. You must provide for this person what you know you would want in his or her place—a compassionate listener. Keep in mind that listening and acknowledging is not the same as agreeing. A person may have done something you feel was not a good idea. You are not agreeing because you choose to listen or acknowledge—you are simply letting the person know you heard and understood what was said.

Every major religion and philosophy in the world makes this point about the need to become more compassionate. If you can become non-judgmental and very compassionate, you're halfway home when it comes to helping people. An added bonus is that you'll make tremendous gains by becoming a more compassionate person.

Golden Rule #3

Do not attempt a diagnosis

How can a person with relatively little training provide emergency help? By not overestimating their role and trying to tell the grieving person what to think about their situation. Just as paramedics don't try to diagnose the condition of their patients, so should people giving emotional first aid not try to diagnose the mental or emotional aspects of the people they help.

Example One:

Alice had experienced the death of her husband and she'd been unable to recover fully from that death even though it happened years ago. Every time she thought of that period of time, the upset surfaced again. Alice had gone through a whole gamut of emotions. She'd been angry, fearful, hostile, and grief stricken. She was able to express the grief but not the anger.

Alice felt that society frowned on a person being angry at a dead spouse and her anger was very strong. She was sure that people would consider it wrong or shameful if they knew how she felt. After all, her husband couldn't help dying. When a compassionate friend helped Alice express the rage, she finally let go of that rage, recognized her emotions for what they were, and recovered from the incident.

Your purpose is to use the questions given in this manual to prompt the traumatized person to talk, and then to listen compassionately and simply acknowledge what you hear. If this sounds like too small a role to be important, then you underestimate greatly the tremendous power of compassionate listening.

Golden Rule #4

Show great interest

There are people who feel others would be offended by great interest or curiosity, and that would be true if the listener was judgmental or critical. We all fear someone probing for our innermost thoughts and feelings and then thinking less of us or criticizing us when they are discovered. Interest is welcomed only when it is coupled with compassion—when we know our confidences are safe and won't be used against us.

Golden Rule #5

Be persistent

When a person finally begins to delve into and talk about their loss and the emotional pain it has caused, it is vital to know that their communication won't be cut short. If you don't have several hours to devote to listening when

> *Example Two:*
>
> *Bill was trying to recover from an addiction. There were times when he had stolen from someone to support his habit and committed a number of other harmful acts. These went against his upbringing and the ethical codes he subscribed to when he was sober, and he thought the crimes were too awful to relate. He was not doing well in his attempts at recovery.*
>
> *When a compassionate friend finally made it possible for him to tell these secrets, he began to make a successful recovery.*

that's what is needed for the person to get through their story completely, it's unwise to start the process. Just as physical first aid measures need to be done completely, so do emotional first aid measures.

The procedures used to help a friend who has just suffered a loss may take half an hour or may take three hours or more—depending on the severity of the loss and the person's willingness and ability to confront it and talk about it. You need to be there for the duration. Each procedure tells how to determine when it has been finished. Always be prepared to take it to that full completion.

Golden Rule #6

Ask simple questions

All the procedures in this book include short, simple, direct questions for you to use to prompt the traumatized person to talk. When a person is undergoing a trauma, simple direct questions are easiest for them to answer.

Golden Rule #7

Acknowledge responses

As people respond to those questions, it is important to let them know they've been heard. A simple "ok" or "uh huh" will suffice. When people aren't sure they've been heard or understood, they may try to explain over and over and become frustrated. Acknowledgments should be simple and unobtrusive—but they are an important part of the process.

Origin of these Golden Rules

These rules were not made up arbitrarily. We all know that there are people who are "naturally" good listeners. These are the people to

The Seven Golden Rules of Emotional First Aid

Be Persistent

Ask Simple Questions

Show Great Interest

Do Not Attempt a Diagnosis

Acknowledge Responses

Listen — Don't Talk

Be Compassionate — Not Critical

whom others instinctively turn when they have a problem to discuss. Even within the professional mental health community, some psychologists, psychiatrists, etc., are known for their natural talent. Those professionals who lack this talent often go into research or teaching rather than having direct client contact. When surveys have been done asking for a description of the qualities most prominent in the people we turn to when we need consolation and help, whether we are discussing professionals or just friends and family, the traits listed in these Golden Rules head the list.

If you take a moment to recall the person you felt most comfortable talking to when you were in trouble, I think you'll find these qualities describe that person well. No amount of professional training will help a critical, judgmental person get good results at rendering emotional first aid. Likewise, professional training will give the naturally compassionate person more techniques and skills to use which increase his or her ability to help others. But even without such training that ability to help will be strong.

Privacy

Discussions that occur as part of the procedures in this book must be treated with the utmost confidentiality. To speak with a friend or acquaintance of the information discussed while using the procedures in this book would be a total betrayal of the person you had tried to help. If you feel you would be unable to grant this degree of confidentiality, don't continue with this book. Send it back for a refund. This is too important a matter to compromise.

Sympathy or Empathy

There is often a misunderstanding about the difference between sympathy and empathy. Empathy requires an understanding of the fact that the other person is in emotional pain. Helping someone try to recover from that pain is the most empathetic action a person can take. Effective help does not require that you sympathize with a person. If you have already sympathized or taken sides in a situation where there is a conflict, it is harder for people to unburden themselves as they may fear that in doing so, your sympathy or support will be eroded. By offering effective help, rather than

sympathy or prejudice, you communicate a non-judgmental attitude that lets the person know your liking for him or her will not
be diminished if you discover that he or she was capable of unwise
actions at times.

Sympathy—as opposed to empathy—is a way of saying that things
really are awful and the person has been truly victimized by what
has happened. There is a place for sympathy, but that place is not
in the hands of the helper. Once again, the similarity between physical and emotional first aid is dramatic. If you were badly injured
in a car accident and required physical therapy to overcome the
resulting disability, would you want a therapist who sympathized
with you or one who effectively got you back on your feet? Would
you want one who spent your precious therapy time agreeing with
you about how awful the drunk driver who hit you was or one who
focused completely on helping you get well?

We have been trained by society to offer sympathy to those who
are grieving. It's time to start offering more. What the grieving
person—child or adult—needs is a compassionate listener who will
help him or her talk at length about the loss; a listener who won't
make him or her wrong for feeling angry or frightened by the loss;
a listener who will steer the mourner to look at those emotions and
decisions experienced at the time of the loss that will have such a
tremendous effect on his or her own life.

Fear of Causing Pain

When you begin using the procedures in this book to apply emotional first aid to your friends or loved ones, your questions will
often result in the person beginning to cry or express distress. This
can be very difficult for you to deal with. Remember the following:
When your child runs in the house with a gash on his or her arm
and you make the decision to use physical first aid to help, one of
the first steps you must take is to wash the injury well to remove
any dirt or germs. This process of cleansing the wound often hurts
and the child may cry. A responsible person does not let the tears
stop him or her from doing what is best for the injury. Not cleaning

the wound may result in infection and a greatly increased recovery time.

The same is true of emotional first aid. Use of the Compassion Remedy in this book is very much equivalent to cleansing a wound. Keep in mind that you are not causing the pain. The injury is causing the pain. Your questions would not produce tears if there was no emotional injury. The only way to stop the pain is to continue the procedure until the person feels the relief of having communicated fully. It takes some courage to help your loved ones emotionally just as it takes courage to clean an injury. Don't let misplaced guilt cause you to back off from offering help.

Blame, Shame, or Regret

Although there are many cases when a trauma or loss is totally caused by an exterior force, like an illness or accident, there are also times when an action taken by the victim made the loss or trauma possible. Therefore it is equally important to make the person comfortable speaking of actions he or she might have taken that contributed to the incident. This is not done in order to assign blame. There is nothing in this Emotional First Aid Manual that is based on blame, shame, or regret. But it is most helpful to address both the areas where one is a victim of the actions of others *and* the areas where one contributed to the situation. Only then can the needed lessons be learned that will help a person avoid a similar problem in the future. The only thing worse than experiencing a certain type of loss once is having it happen more than once because the lessons that help avoid it weren't learned.

Goals for Emotional First Aid

It is important to recognize that your goal in helping someone recover from any trauma or loss will not result in the person instantly recovering ompletely and becoming totally happy. Just as when physical first aid is used, the result of your efforts doesn't mean the injury is instantly and miraculously healed. It does mean that your efforts to do the equivalent of cleansing the wound to prevent infection and applying a healing salve will result in the person being able to move smoothly through the natural recovery period for that type of injury.

You may occasionally achieve complete relief with a more minor loss or trauma, but with a serious trauma like a death, that is an unrealistic goal. What you can do is help the person move freely and more rapidly through the stages of grief on their way to a full recovery. Sadly, it is not uncommon for a person to get hung up in one of the stages and spend years suffering because of it. Being unable to communicate fully about a trauma is equivalent to having a physical wound become infected and it results in a much longer recovery period and sometimes prevents recovery completely. This is the reason why some people recover within a relatively short period of time while others are still suffering years later. Someone who receives help from a compassionate listener will recover from the feeling of terrible loss much more rapidly than someone who doesn't receive such help. This does not mean a person won't still miss someone or something that they lost. It means they will more rapidly be able to recover, move on with life, and be able to once again experience moments of great happiness. It also means the person will be more likely to learn any life lessons available as a result of the event and therefore reduce the possibility of a similar loss or trauma happening again.

How to Use this Book

Like a physical first aid manual, this book does not need to be read straight through. It is very important to read the Foreword, Introduction, and this Vital Information section before you try to provide emotional first aid. It is also useful to read the introduction to each of the book's sections so you have an overview of the subject of emotional first aid. It is not necessary for you to read about every type of trauma in the book before beginning to use the procedures. The table of contents will help you find the subject matter that applies to a specific person you might want to help. Before you begin to offer that help, it is best to refresh your memory by rereading this Vital Information section and then reading the part of the book that gives specific instructions about the type of trauma you will be addressing.

Frequently Asked Questions

Below are some of the questions asked most frequently by those who are new to the application of the remedies in this book:

Q. How do I know whether I can be successful doing these procedures?

A. Are you a good listener or are you willing to learn to be one? That is the single most important trait necessary for an emotional first aid provider. It also helps if you have a genuine interest in people and a curiosity about how the mind works. You do not have to be brilliant or highly educated but you do need to be able to recognize the importance of the Golden Rules of Emotional First Aid and be willing to follow them.

Q. How do I approach someone who appears to be suffering from a trauma?

A. While it can vary from one situation to another, an easy way to determine that is by looking at the physical first aid model. If you saw someone lying on the pavement bleeding, your first reaction would be to call for professional help if the injury looked severe. Then you might do what you could to apply your knowledge of first aid by applying pressure to stem the bleeding and making sure the person was as comfortable as possible while waiting for the professional help to arrive. In an extremely severe case, you might need to use CPR to keep the person alive until the help arrived. If the injury looked more minor or if professional help was not available, you might let the person know that you have had some training in first aid procedures and ask them if they would like you to clean and bandage the wound.

Venting strong negative emotions can be the equivalent of bleeding in the emotional first aid case. A person who is crying or visibly angry or extremely agitated is emotionally bleeding. A person who has all emotions suppressed may be the equivalent of the unconscious physical first aid case. When you know someone has suffered a terrible loss but their emotions seem to be frozen, it is best to encourage them to get professional help because they are likely to be very difficult for the layperson to help. But if they are visibly crying, angry, agitated or otherwise upset, you may be able to help them and you can say just that. Often you don't even need to do more than say, "How are you doing?" in an empathetic tone of voice and the floodgates open and the person genuinely starts telling you.

Q. How soon after a loss should I offer help?

A. With a death, the first week or two after the event, the person is surrounded by friends and loved ones and is very focused on handling things like arrangements for a memorial service or insurance matters. You can use the Calming Procedure (see index for page location) right away to help them through the first few days. But a week or two after the loss, often they are alone and would really welcome some company. Try to visit when you will have enough time and privacy to provide them with sufficient help and then invite them to talk about how they are doing. You will usually find it very easy to help a person at that point.

Use similar judgment with other types of traumas. If you can schedule a visit when the person will have sufficient time and privacy to talk, that is always best. In the case of a child who comes home from school crying because they have suffered a traumatic event, acting immediately is best if possible. The sooner the better is a good rule of thumb but realistically, it may take a week or two before an opportunity presents itself, especially with adults. It is never too late. When a person had suffered the trauma even years earlier but still is suffering the effects, he or she can still be helped.

Conclusion

These are the absolute basics on which all of the technology in this manual will be based. If someone received no other training at all but learned to be a little more compassionate, show a little more interest, and have a little more persistence and patience, that person would have increased tremendously his or her ability to help someone. If you get nothing else out of this manual then what we've just covered, that alone would stand you in good stead. It would make you better able to help your friends, your children, and your acquaintances.

Introduction to Section One

When it comes to spending your valuable time helping a friend or loved one, you have two choices; offering that person sympathy—or offering that person effective help. This book is about ways to offer effective help.

What is the hardest part of helping someone who has just experienced the adultery of a spouse, the loss of a job, the betrayal of a friend, or any of the other traumas our lives can include? Resisting the impulse to sympathize or take sides!

Why must you resist it? Sympathy (as opposed to empathy or compassion) and prejudice are not compatible with effective help. Sympathy and prejudice are a form of agreement that things are awful and the person has been victimized. It's not that sympathy has no place in the world, but that place is not as a facet of the role of delivering effective emotional first aid.

Example:

Tom was badly injured in a car accident when he was struck by a drunk driver. Extensive rehabilitation was needed to restore his ability to walk. Tom had two primary therapists: Helen and Astrid. He paid over $100 per hour for both therapy sessions.

Helen spent at least 15 minutes of every session sympathizing with Tom over the injuries and going on about the horrors of drunk driving. The things she said were true and Tom enjoyed having someone understand his feelings.

Astrid, on the other hand, got right down to business and drove Tom to push himself to the limits to make his rehabilitation complete. She was not as sympathetic as Helen but she showed compassion by working tirelessly to bring about Tom's recovery.

Eventually Tom realized that the gains he made in his sessions with Astrid far outweighed those made in his sessions with Helen. As he began to see a full recovery in sight he also came to understand the difference between compassion and sympathy.

Compassion is not always "nice". On the contrary, Astrid had often been irritating in her demands for more and more effort from Tom. But Astrid's actions were always based on her desire to see Tom fully recovered. She had a true understanding of the unhappiness Tom would continue to feel if he went through life permanently disabled. Tom realized that the short-term pleasure of having someone sympathize with his pain and agree with his anger was far outweighed by the long-term pleasure of becoming whole again.

The procedures you will do in this book can sometimes seem grueling and unsympathetic. Asking a friend or loved one to tell you again about a terrible trauma in his or her life when doing so causes tears to flow and pain to be re-experienced is not for the fainthearted. If you are persistent and follow the procedures to their completion without violating the Golden Rules of Emotional First Aid (found in the Chapter titled Vital Information), then you will have the pleasure of helping that loved one become whole again. Nothing can top that experience for either of you.

There are four distinct phases a person goes through when he/she experiences a trauma. How much time is spent in each phase is determined largely by the quality of the help received by that person. The four stages are as follows:

Shock

Trauma victims may feel dazed or immobilized at times, have difficulty with their memory, or feel as though their sense of time is distorted. They are likely to feel angry, anxious, and frustrated. Physical reactions like nausea, muscle aches, and a pounding heart are common with emotional trauma.

Denial

Trauma victims may begin to doubt what they saw and that it had any effect upon them. They may feel emotionally numb and wish to isolate themselves from co-workers, family and friends, or conversely be euphoric or "wired" and want to talk.

Impact

The full impact of the incident begins to sink in after the initial shock and denial have subsided. Often people have nightmares following a trauma and most have a difficult time sleeping for at least a few days. Trauma victims might feel preoccupied with thoughts about it during the day. In very strong trauma, brief lapses can occur when the person feels as if the incident is actually reoccurring. These "mini-flashbacks" can be particularly disturbing, and can make victims feel as if they are going crazy. They are not. These are all normal responses to abnormal events and should improve over time. Trauma victims may also question how well they performed during the disaster. They may condemn themselves—or others—for not doing enough or obsess about "what if...." These self-doubts are common and expected. They are also very often exaggerated or unfounded. It's important for victims not to give in to such feelings of self-blame, rage, or depression by isolating themselves or using drugs, alcohol, or other substances to cope. This will only make things worse.

Resolution

Recovery from psychological traumatization is a painful, but natural process for most people. It is normal for anyone who has been psychologically traumatized to need to talk about what happened—to co-workers, family, friends, clergy, counselors, etc. Especially valuable are talks with people who have been through the same thing or something similar. They can understand what the trauma victim is experiencing. This is the reason support groups can be so helpful. The more the person talks about it with people who understand, the sooner the difficulties will pass.

When the trauma victim has some understanding of what the phases entail, it can be easier for him or her to deal with the trauma. It is important for people to know that they are not alone in their feelings and are not going crazy, but are having perfectly normal reactions. One of the techniques you will learn in this book is called an Orientation Remedy. It is designed to be done right at the scene of the trauma if necessary and it includes the information above as an educational step. Because it would be difficult to memorize these materials, the most basic procedure, the Compassion Remedy, is provided in the book on a removable card that you can carry with you.

In addition to the procedures listed in each section of this book, there are actions that can be taken in life to help someone who has been traumatized. These actions are referred to as the Calming Procedure. Do as many of these actions as it is possible for you to do.

- ❐ Help create a calm, quiet, predictable environment for the traumatized person

- ❐ Encourage the person to get extra nutritional support (stress burns more nutrients)

- ❐ Treat the person as gently as possible recognizing that an emotional injury is as destructive as a physical one

- ❐ Give as much physical contact as appropriate and acceptable: hugs, hand holding, pats on the shoulder, etc.

- ❐ Be reassuring whenever possible

- ❐ Help provide the presence of a compassionate person until the worst of the trauma has passed

- ❐ Provide as much unconditional love as you can

- ❐ Do the appropriate procedures from the sections of this book that follow

Don't be afraid to try to help! If you are motivated by a desire to help and follow the few simple rules in the Chapter called Vital Information, you certainly will do no harm, and you may have the joy of helping a loved one to a full recovery!

Section One—Adult Trauma

Loss of a Job

The loss of a job is often underestimated in its potential for devastating effects on a person's life. While the occasional individual takes it lightly (usually someone with a large bank account and good prospects for immediate re-employment), most of us rate it right up there with a divorce or a serious accident when it comes to overall stress. The reasons for this are numerous and include damage to ego and sense of self-worth, the threat of financial ruin, the loss of friendships and close ties, and the necessity of confronting potential rejection in the search for a new position. Never take lightly the effects of job loss even when the person is putting up a brave front. Many people find it hard to talk even to friends and family about such a loss because of the damage to their self-esteem.

Because medical insurance and regular paychecks often come to an end with the job, the unemployed person who is suffering depression or great upset is unlikely to seek professional help. His or her need for comfort from friends and family is usually at an all-time high.

Pep talks are tempting ways to try to help a friend but they are rarely effective, giving only a short-term boost at best. No matter how reasonable a person tries to be, losing a job can cut right to the core of his or her self esteem. Unless you are the last person fired or laid off before the company shuts its doors, a job termination creates the idea that you are expendable, that you aren't worth the salary you were being paid.

Because this often causes the newly unemployed person to feel strong emotions that are not "acceptable" in society, emotions like anger, bitterness, resentment, and fear, it can be difficult to get the person to open up and express those emotions.

If you truly want to help someone who has suffered a job loss, you will need to be prepared to follow the Seven Golden Rules of Emotional First Aid scrupulously. If you haven't recently read the chapter called Vital Information, be sure to do so again. Compassionate, non-judgmental communication will be the key to helping the person express those unacceptable emotions and thus get relief from them.

The best way to build confidence in order to get a new job is to communicate those feelings fully. The procedure that follows is designed to help you help your loved one open up and express himself or herself. Be prepared to spend as much time as needed. There are times when the person has had a string of job losses and the procedure below will need to be done on several of them beginning with the most recent and continuing backwards in time. It is best also to start at the very beginning of the job loss. This part of the incident might be when the person first began to suspect there might be trouble months before the actual termination occurred.

On rare occasions, a person is reluctant to begin speaking of the loss. In that case, begin a conversation about the job he or she just

> **Example**
>
> *When Denise lost her job unexpectedly, she told all her friends she was glad because she had hated her boss anyway. But after several months she still had no prospects for another job and was drinking more than usual, sleeping late every day, and avoiding her friends. A wise friend realized it was possible to feel a loss even over a job that was hated.*
>
> *In the course of using the Compassion Remedy on Denise, her friend discovered the problem went all the way back to the first job Denise had ever held. She had loved that job and been shocked when it suddenly ended. At that time, she had decided it wasn't smart to get too attached to any job because it only set you up for a loss eventually. Although that decision had seemed to protect her from further loss, it had also kept Denise from much of the pleasure that can be obtained through a career.*
>
> *On inspection of the moment she had made this decision and the effects it had on her life, Denise decided that she would rather risk a future loss than lose all her pleasure in work. With her improved attitude and relief from much of the grief she had felt, Denise found it easier to continue her job search and she found a position she liked in a short time.*

held and what it was like, and quite naturally, when the person begins to feel more comfortable with you, he or she will progress to speaking of the termination.

Now begin the Compassion Remedy that follows:

Compassion Remedy

The first step in handling a recent loss or trauma is to encourage the person to talk about it and to listen carefully to what the person says. Some encouragement may be needed at first. You can encourage a person to say more by use of the following prompts:

1. Tell me what happened.

2. Did anything else happen.'

3. Is there anything else you want to tell me about that?

"When did you first realize there might be a loss of your job in the future?" is also a useful prompt. At no time during the conversation should you become critical or judgmental. Make a point of always letting the person know that you have heard what he or she is saying. A simple "uh huh" or "ok" is enough to acknowledge that you have heard someone. Most people will be very eager to talk to you as long as you remain compassionate and interested. You encourage the person to communicate fully by avoiding judgmental or critical communication or attitudes and by following the Golden Rules of Emotional First Aid. The person's recounting of the event may run for a few minutes or several hours. Be prepared to listen patiently throughout. If the person has told you about the incident but still has attention on it, ask him or her to tell you about it again one or more times.

Frequently, after telling you about the event, the person feels relieved and has no further interest in the event. If that is the case, end the Compassion Remedy at that point. If that is not the case, ask the person if there is something he or she now feels could be done about the event or if he or she now sees some way to handle the effects of the event in a positive manner. Looking at this point of view may help the person feel able to act as cause in the event rather than feeling victimized by it.

It is also important to check with the person for any decisions he or she might have made at the time of the incident. Often a person makes major decisions during a time of loss and it is beneficial to take note of those decisions and to talk about them to a friend. Sometimes the decisions were wise ones and the talk reinforces them, but there are other times when the decisions would have proved to be destructive. An example might be someone who decides never to risk trying for an important job again because the loss was so painful. If left unexamined, that decision could prove to be harmful. Once the person has had the chance to talk about the loss at length and to begin the healing process, he or she might change his or her mind about the wisdom of such a decision. The spotting of decisions and communication about them with a compassionate listener is one of the most beneficial parts of this procedure. There may be one decision or many. Take plenty of time on this question and give the person the chance to examine all decisions.

If, during the course of doing this procedure, the person starts to speak of an earlier similar job loss, go ahead and ask the person to focus on that earlier time and ask the same series of questions about that incident.

When all decisions made at that earliest time have been viewed, the person will feel relieved and more extroverted and it is then time to end the procedure.

It can take some time for the process of grieving to come to a closure.

If you feel the reactions of your friend or loved one to the incident are extreme, use the list of resources at the end of this section to encourage professional help. For the person who has strong ties to a religious group, there is often pastoral counseling available. For those who don't, many wonderful counseling centers exist where help can be obtained. The appendix of this book contains references to help find professional help.

Loss of Hopes and Dreams

The loss of a hope or dream is often part of another loss. The break-up of a marriage, for instance, also involves the loss of the dream of a happy union. The loss of a child also involves the loss of all your dreams for that child. But there are also losses of hopes or dreams that stand alone.

The dream of living in peace can be crushed by the onset of war. The dream of becoming a dancer can be crushed by the day-to-day rejections of a tough business or by a sudden physical injury or the accumulation of many small injuries. A sudden feeling of loss of a hope or dream is easier to spot in another person. There is a dramatic change following the realization of the loss.

Gradual losses may be harder to spot. Here are some clues that will help you tell when your friends or loved ones have suffered such a loss.

- a general drop in emotional level (cheerful to apathetic, for example)
- a visible drop in brightness/alertness
- frequent illness in a formerly healthy person
- an increased need for sleep
- an increase in drinking and/or drug use
- a sharp increase or decrease in consumption of food

If you have a friend or loved one who has been excited about plans for the future—goals or dreams—and you observe a fall off in that excitement, don't wait! The time to offer a compassionate ear is before he or she becomes totally discouraged. Whether the loss is due to a series of small rejections or one big one, the method for helping is similar.

There are people who give up on a dream that could have been turned to reality if they had only been able to persist a little longer. Your help might enable them to stay with in the face of rejection and ultimately win.

Other times, the dream was not possible, at least not in the exact way the person saw it. An example might be someone who dreamed of a happy relationship with his or her current spouse. The fulfillment of that dream requires the efforts of both parties. For that reason, the person does not have full control over the outcome and can fail through no fault of his or her own. Your help might enable that person to give up the dream of having a good relationship with that one specific unwilling person and yet succeed ultimately at the broader goal of having a happy relationship with a willing partner. Thus, your intention in helping is not to insist that the person continue toward the exact same dream but to see him or her regain confidence

---

Example

Tom had always dreamed of playing professional baseball. When he was dropped from a minor-league team, he felt the end of his dreams had come. He was twenty-six years old by then and younger players were moving up while he fell behind.

A friend was able to get him to talk about his dreams of being a big-league player. It was painful to listen as it was clear Tom was not going to be able to bounce back. His body had suffered too many injuries and, although he was a fantastic player compared to most of us, he lacked the extreme physical attributes needed to be at the top of the game. It would have been easy to just feel sorry for Tom but his friend persisted in encouraging him to look all the way back to the first time he had ever dreamed of being a star player.

When Tom spotted the fact that the birth of his dream occurred while watching a professional game with his father, he realized that some of the reason he felt so devastated by the loss of the dream was that he felt it was the only way he could have gained the admiration of his father who was an ardent baseball fan. With that long buried decision opened up, he was able to realize that he had earned his father's respect and that life could still be pleasurable whether he made it to the big leagues or not.

---

and either strengthen his or her resolve to attain the original dream or recognize the need to broaden the dream and work toward attaining that.

If you haven't recently read the chapter titled Vital Information, reread it now and then proceed with the following information.

Compassion Remedy

The first step in handling a recent loss or trauma is to encourage the person to talk about it and to listen carefully to what the person says. Some encouragement may be needed at first. You can encourage a person to say more by use of the following prompts:

1. Tell me what happened.

2. Did anything else happen?

3. Is there anything else you want to tell me about that?

"When did you first realize there might be a loss of your dream in the future?" is also a useful prompt. At no time during the conversation should you become critical or judgmental. Make a point of always letting the person know that you have heard what he or she is saying. A simple "uh huh" or "ok" is enough to acknowledge that you have heard someone. Most people will be very eager to talk to you as long as you remain compassionate and interested. You encourage the person to communicate fully by avoiding judgmental or critical communication or attitudes and by following the Golden Rules of Emotional First Aid. The person's recounting of the event may run for a few minutes or several hours. Be prepared to listen patiently throughout. If the person has told you about the incident but still has attention on it, ask him or her to tell you about it again one or more times. When a series of smaller rejections over a period of many years is involved rather than one shorter large rejection, it can still be treated as one incident. Ask how long the person has been trying to obtain this dream and then let him or her know that you want to hear about that entire time period.

Frequently, after telling you about the event, the person feels relieved and has no further interest in the event. If that is the case, end the Compassion Remedy at that point. If that is not the case, ask the person if there is something he or she now feels could be done about the event or if he or she now sees some way to handle the effects of the event in a positive manner. Looking at this point of view may help the person feel able to act as cause in the event rather than feeling victimized by it.

Check also for any decisions the person might have made at the time of the incident. Often a person makes major decisions during a time of loss and it is beneficial to take note of those decisions and to talk about them to a friend. Sometimes the decisions were wise ones and the talk reinforces them, but there are other times when the decisions would have proved to be destructive. An example might be someone who decides never to try to attain his or her dreams again. If left unexamined, that decision could prove to be harmful. Once the person has had the chance to talk about the loss at length and to begin the healing process, he or she might change his or her mind about the wisdom of such a decision. The spotting of decisions and communication about them with a compassionate listener is one of the most beneficial parts of this procedure. There may be one decision or many. Take plenty of time on this question and give the person the chance to examine all decisions.

If, during the course of doing this procedure, the person starts to speak of an earlier similar loss of a hope or dream, go ahead and focus on that earlier time and ask the same series of questions about that incident.

When all decisions made at that earliest time have been viewed, the person will feel relieved and more extroverted and it is then time to end the procedure.

In the rare event that the person doesn't want to talk about the end of the dream, encourage him or her to talk about the dream itself, and when the person becomes more comfortable talking to you, he or she will quite naturally begin to speak of the end of the dream.

If you feel the reactions of your friend or loved one to the incident are extreme, use the list of resources in the appendix to encourage professional help. For the person who has ties to a religious group, there is often pastoral counseling available. For those who don't, many wonderful counseling centers exist where help can be obtained. The appendix contains references to find professional help.

Trauma of Feeling Different

Feeling "different" can be enjoyable when the difference is one we have chosen, but when that difference is forced upon us by circumstances, we may react quite differently. The loss here is based on a desire most people have to be "normal" or like their peers or people they admire. The part of the situation that is traumatic begins with the first moment the person decides he or she is different and that it is undesirable to be different. The person who never notices his or her differences or who never sees it as a negative condition will not need help in this area. The person who is aware of a perceived difference and dislikes it may need a great deal of help.

In an ideal world, we would all accept and appreciate our own differences and those of our fellow men and there would be no loss attached to it. But this is far from being an ideal world.

How can you tell when a person does need help in this area? Look for some of the following signs:

- Dressing to hide a physical difference (Example: wearing long sleeves even in the warmest weather to cover a birthmark or scar.)

- Avoiding certain activities because they might show off a physical difference (Example: an overweight person who won't participate in sports but looks wistfully on from the sidelines.)

- Avoiding activities like games because they might reveal a lack of mental quickness or agility

Ultimately we want our loved ones to have the strength to deal with a difference; not to simply conform at all cost. Making a person wrong for caring about a difference is not the answer however. Encouraging the friend or loved one to communicate fully about his or her feelings of being different is the answer.

People often make life changing decisions based on such an upset and those changes can be destructive. We need to allow all the emotion to be voiced and the decisions made to be re-examined. By doing this, we help a friend or loved one learn not to allow his or her life to be destroyed by these differences. It is vital on this procedure to find the moment when the person first decided that they were different from others and that they felt it was a negative difference.

Compassion Remedy

The first step in handling a recent loss or trauma is to encourage the person to talk about it and to listen carefully to what the person says. Some encouragement may be needed at first. You can encourage a person to say more by use of the following prompts:

1. Tell me what happened.

2. Did anything else happen?

3. Is there anything else you want to tell me about that?

Example

Jim had suffered a brain injury in his youth that caused him to process information more slowly. When, during a card game, a girlfriend had made fun of him for thinking slowly, it set him on a lifetime pattern of avoiding games of all sorts. Even though his wife and children would never have thought less of him and would have enjoyed having him join in the fun, Jim couldn't bring himself to participate in their activities.

It wasn't until a friend who was an excellent listener became curious about why Jim wouldn't participate and asked him about it that Jim finally realized how much his decision to avoid the possibility of humiliation had cost him. After talking it out, he realized that there were some situations where it was safe to enjoy games with people who were not critical or impatient.

At no time during the conversation should you become critical or judgmental. Make a point of always letting the person know that you have heard what he or she is saying. A simple "uh huh" or "ok" is enough to acknowledge that you have heard someone. Most people will be very eager to talk to you as long as you remain compassionate and interested. You encourage the person to communicate fully by avoiding judgmental or critical communication or attitudes and by following the Golden Rules of Emotional First Aid. The person's recounting of the event may run for a few minutes or several hours. Be prepared to listen patiently throughout. If the person has told you about the incident but still has attention on it, ask him or her to tell you about it again one or more times.

Frequently, after telling you about the event, the person feels relieved and has no further interest in the event. If that is the case, end the Compassion Remedy at that point. If that is not the case, ask the person if there is something he or she now feels could be done about the event or if he or she now sees some way to handle the effects of the event in a positive manner. Looking at this point of view may help the person feel able to act as cause in the event rather than feeling victimized by it.

Check also for any decisions the person might have made at the time of the incident. Often someone makes major decisions during a time of stress and it is beneficial to take note of those decisions and to talk about them to a friend or loved one. Sometimes the decisions were wise ones and the talk reinforces them, but there are other times when the decisions would have proved to be destructive. An example might be a person who decides he or she is worthless because of his or her differences. If left unexamined, that decision could prove to be harmful. Once the person has had the chance to talk about the upset at length and to begin the healing process, that person might change his or her mind about the wisdom of such a decision. The spotting of decisions and communication about them with a compassionate listener is one of the most beneficial parts of this procedure. There may be one decision or many. Take plenty of time on this question and give the person the chance to examine all decisions.

If, during the course of doing this procedure, the person starts to speak of an earlier similar upset, go ahead and ask the person to examine that earlier time and ask the same series of questions about that incident.

When all decisions made at that earliest time have been viewed, the person will feel relieved and more extroverted and it is then time to end the procedure.

If you feel the reactions of your friend or loved one to the incident are extreme, use the list of resources in the appendix to encourage professional help. For the person who has strong ties to a religious group, there is often pastoral counseling available. For those who don't, many wonderful counseling centers exist where help can be obtained. The appendix of the book contains references to help find professional help.

Trauma of Feeling like a Disappointment

There is a very destructive technique used by some people to try to gain control over the behavior of others. It's called, *"You're such a disappointment to me."* By saying this with the "proper" tone of voice, the controlling person hopes to manipulate a vulnerable person (often a child) into meeting the controlling person's standards or working toward the controlling person's goals. A life spent working to achieve someone else's goals will not be a rewarding lifetime.

When this technique is used by someone for whom you have little respect, love, or admiration, it's easy to shrug it off and see the attempt to manipulate for what it is. But when it's used by someone you do care for, it can be quite devastating. Is there anything that feels worse? Yes! It's deciding that you have disappointed yourself.

Is telling someone they have disappointed you ever a positive technique that will cause that person to abandon destructive behavior in favor of more constructive behavior? No! There are much better ways to encourage someone to adopt more pro-survival behavior. If you can't think of any, turn to the appendix in the back of the book for some suggestions on classes or reading material that will aid you in finding a more productive way of encouraging others. Making someone feel like a disappointment will only cause a loss of self esteem and a resulting drop in the constructiveness of his or her behavior.

How can you tell when a friend or loved one is suffering from the feeling of being a disappointment to themselves or others? The symptoms are not hard to spot. They include the following:

- A sudden drop in the person's emotional level (from cheerfulness to grief, for example)

- An air of hopelessness

- A tendency to cry easily

- The giving-up of activities formerly enjoyed

- A sudden sense of shame or embarrassment

There are a number of problems that can cause similar symptoms so it's important, when you see the signs above in a friend or loved one, to encourage them to talk in a general way about how life is going. Then watch for any statement that shows a feeling that they have been a disappointment to others. If you have turned to this chapter in this Emotional First Aid Manual instinctively, then the loved one's comments have probably already communicated to you that this is the help needed. If you aren't certain, there is no harm in asking the person if someone has made them feel like a disappointment. If yes, proceed with the remedy below. If not, continue the conversation until you are able to determine, by listening closely, just which of the sections in this book would apply.

> **Example**
>
> *Susan was a nurturing, caring individual who chose to work in the child-care field because it was so emotionally rewarding. The salaries in that field are far less than they should be but Susan felt the emotional rewards were far more important as she pursued her goal of earning a degree in early childhood education. She was feeling very pleased until her father, a man she loved and respected and a highly successful business-man, expressed his disappointment that she had not chosen a profession that would pay well and "make her successful" like he was. Although she tried to explain why she wanted the career she had chosen, her father could not see past the financial side of the picture.*
>
> *While her father meant well and simply wanted to make sure his daughter would never face financial difficulties, his expression of disappointment in her choices had a very damaging effect on her. Some of the joy in her career was gone and Susan began to feel less confident about her future. When she received some emotional first aid for the loss of confidence, she realized that she could reassure her father that she would not put herself in actual financial danger and maintain her love for him without letting his disappointment erode her self-confidence.*

When you are certain the problem is that the person feels they are a disappointment, use the Compassion Remedy to help.

Compassion Remedy

The first step in handling a recent loss or trauma is to encourage the person to talk about it and to listen carefully to what the person says. Some encouragement may be needed at first. You can encourage a person to say more by use of the following prompts:

1. Tell me what happened.

2. Did anything else happen?

3. Is there anything else you want to tell me about that?

At no time during the conversation should you become critical or judgmental. Make a point of always letting the person know that you have heard what he or she is saying. A simple "uh huh" or "ok" is enough to acknowledge that you have heard someone. Most people will be very eager to talk to you as long as you remain compassionate and interested. You encourage the person to communicate fully by avoiding judgmental or critical communication or attitudes and by following the Golden Rules of Emotional First Aid. The person's recounting of the event may run for a few minutes or several hours. Be prepared to listen patiently throughout. If the person has told you about the incident but still has attention on it, ask him or her to tell you about it again one or more times.

Frequently, after telling you about the event, the person feels relieved and has no further interest in the event. If that is the case, end the Compassion Remedy at that point. If that is not the case, ask the person if there is something he or she now feels could be done about the event or if he or she now sees some way to handle the effects of the event in a positive manner. Looking at this point of view may help the person feel able to act as cause in the event rather than feeling victimized by it.

Check also for any decisions the person might have made at the time of the incident. Often a person makes major decisions during a time of loss and it is beneficial to take note of those decisions and to talk about them to a friend. Sometimes the decisions were wise ones and the talk reinforces them, but there are other times when the decisions would have proved to be destructive. An example might be someone who decides always to try to be what others want him to be so he will never disappoint anyone again. If left unexamined, that decision could prove to be harmful. Once the person has had the chance to talk about the loss at length and to begin the healing process, he or she might change his or her mind about the wisdom of such a decision. The spotting of decisions and communication about them with a compassionate listener is one of the most beneficial parts of this procedure. There may be one decision or many. Take plenty of time on this question and give the person the chance to examine all decisions.

If, during the course of doing this procedure, the person starts to speak of an earlier similar time when he or she felt like a disappointment, go ahead and ask the person to examine that earlier time and ask the same series of questions about that incident.

When all decisions made at that earliest time have been viewed, the person will feel relieved and more extroverted and it is then time to end the procedure.

If you feel the reactions of your friend or loved one to the incident are extreme, use the list of resources in the appendix to encourage professional help. For the person who has strong ties to a religious group, there is often pastoral counseling available. For those who don't, many wonderful counseling centers exist where help can be obtained. The appendix contains references to help find professional help.

Trauma of Failure to Help Someone

A strong desire to help another person is admirable, but when it does not succeed, it can result in one of the heaviest losses a person can experience. Examples of this are everywhere: the parents who try to help a gravely ill child; a spouse who tries to help a partner with a terminal illness or an addiction; the caretaker for a person who is seriously mentally ill. All of these are examples of situations where help is difficult to provide and often fails. The most extreme example may be the sense of failure experienced by loved ones of a person who commits suicide. There is often a long period of attempts to help preceding the suicide and a tremendous feeling of loss when the help does not prevent the tragedy.

Example

Alice was suffering from terminal cancer. Her husband saw no way to help her as the disease progressed rapidly throughout her body. Although he performed many of the caretaking tasks, he did not consider those to be of real help since she was still dying. Nothing Alice said could convince him his help was very real and valuable.

When Alice finally realized she needed to stop doing the talking and trying to coax him into realizing he was helping her, she started to listen and ask him questions. Using the techniques in the Compassion Remedy, she encouraged him to tell her about all his feelings of failure to help. It was hard for Alice to listen to this. She wanted to interrupt and convince him he was helping but she stifled the urge and followed the procedure.

When she finally checked to see if there was an earlier time in his life when he felt he had failed to help, he began to tell her of an experience in his childhood when he had felt helpless in dealing with his mother's depression. As he recounted his feelings at that time, he finally realized he had made some serious decisions during his mother's illness. He had concluded that he lacked the ability to be useful and decided there was something very wrong with him.

Once Alice's husband communicated fully about this incident, he was able to see that, while he couldn't prevent his wife's death, he was truly able to help her.

When you see a friend or loved one suffering such a loss, remember that the helper is sometimes in need of help too. And the best help you can offer someone is a compassionate listener. We would all like to do more. We'd like to just be able to make the problem go away. It's often not possible. But never underestimate the help you can provide. It's quite common, when you are offering a compassionate ear to someone who fits the examples given above, for that person to realize that he or she did not totally fail to help either. It might seem that we've failed to help the terminally ill person when he or she dies, but the time we spent listening to that person's fears may have been successful help in every sense of the word.

People who work in the "caregiving/helping" professions, doctors, nurses, therapists, social workers, ministers, etc., should have their own needs addressed regularly so that the occasional failures they experience do not drive them down the scale of emotions. There must be a special place in Heaven for those who help the "helpers". There is no one more deserving of help than the person who has been beaten down by their feeling of failure in attempts to help another. Don't stand by and watch it happen. The procedure that follows will do much to restore the morale and confidence of the discouraged helper.

Compassion Remedy

The first step in handling a recent loss or trauma is to encourage the person to talk about it and to listen carefully to what the person says. Some encouragement may be needed at first. You can encourage a person to say more by use of the following prompts:

1. Tell me what happened.

2. Did anything else happen?

3. Is there anything else you want to tell me about that?

At no time during the conversation should you become critical or judgmental. Make a point of always letting the person know that you have heard what he or she is saying. A simple "uh huh" or "ok" is enough to acknowledge that you have heard someone. Most people will be very eager to talk to you as long as you remain compassionate and interested. You encourage the person to communicate fully by avoiding judgmental or critical communication or attitudes and by following the Golden Rules of Emotional First Aid. The person's recounting of the event may run for a few minutes or several hours. Be prepared to listen patiently throughout. If the person has told you about the incident but still has attention on it, ask him or her to tell you about it again one or more times.

Frequently, after telling you about the event, the person feels relieved and has no further interest in the event. If that is the case, end the Compassion Remedy at that point. If that is not the case, ask the person if there is something he or she now feels could be done about the event or if he or she now sees some way to handle the effects of the event in a positive manner. Looking at this point of view may help the person feel able to act as cause in the event rather than feeling victimized by it.

Check also for any decisions the person might have made at the time of the incident. Often a person makes major decisions during a time of loss and it is beneficial to take note of those decisions and to talk about them to a friend. Sometimes the decisions were wise ones and the talk reinforces them, but there are other times when the decisions would have proved to be destructive. An example might be someone who decides to give up helping others so he or she will never be hurt again. If left unexamined, that decision could prove to be harmful. Once the person has had the chance to talk about the loss at length and to begin the healing process, he or she might change his or her mind about the wisdom of such a decision. The spotting of decisions and communication about them with a compassionate listener is one of the most beneficial parts of this procedure. There may be one decision or many. Take plenty of time on this question and give the person the chance to examine all decisions.

If, during the course of doing this procedure, the person starts to speak of an earlier similar time when he or she felt a failure to help, go ahead and ask the person to examine that earlier time and ask the same series of questions about that incident.

When all decisions made at that earliest time have been viewed, the person will feel relieved and more extroverted and it is then time to end the procedure.

If you feel the reactions of your friend or loved one to the incident are extreme, use the list of resources in the appendix to encourage professional help. For the person who has strong ties to a religious group, there is often pastoral counseling available. For those who don't, many wonderful counseling centers exist where help can be obtained. The appendix of the book contains references to help find professional help.

Loss through Divorce, Separation, or Abandonment

Helping a friend or loved one who is facing or going through a divorce, separation, or abandonment is not an easy task. Whether the person instigates the action or is an unwilling participant, he or she will still be feeling a huge array of emotions, many of them conflicting.

There are two key things for the helper to keep in mind. Sympathy is not an effective way to help; good communication skills and a compassionate ear are the keys to aiding your friends or loved ones. Taking sides in the action is also of no real value, no matter how much you may feel your friend has been wronged.

Divorces, separations, and abandonments are rarely completely one sided in terms of constructive or destructive actions by the parties involved. Often, in the course of communicating openly and freely about the situation to a friend, a spouse will find it helpful to unburden himself or herself about the things he or she may have done that he or she now regrets.

Example

Tom and Sally were getting a divorce. It was a shock to all their friends who had not seen it coming. It was a shock to Tom also because he had thought the marriage, while it wasn't perfect, was worth continuing.

When Tom's minister, Bob, tried to help Tom overcome his grief and bitterness, Tom had a hard time being honest with him. Although Sally had entered into an affair and it was easy to blame her for the divorce, Tom had done some things he felt ashamed of including criticizing Sally frequently for her shortcomings.

Tom felt some relief in being able to talk to Bob about how betrayed and angry he felt but that alone did not provide the relief he needed. When Bob was finally able to encourage Tom to discuss the things he had done that he now regretted, Tom began to feel a greater sense of relief. He was able to see that he needed to handle his tendency to be critical or future relationships would also fail. Although the marriage could not be salvaged, it was vital for the sake of the children that Tom and Sally have a cooperative attitude where their children were concerned. When Tom was able to look at his own contributions to the failure of the relationship, he became more confident that he could get over the loss and take steps to ensure that his future relationships would work.

If you have already sympathized or taken sides, it is harder for the person to do this unburdening as he or she may fear that in doing so, your sympathy or support will be eroded. By offering effective help, rather than sympathy or prejudice, you communicate a non-judgmental attitude that lets the person know your liking for him or her will not be diminished if you discover he or she was capable of unwise actions at times.

The key to help in this situation is to make it very safe for the person to discuss not only the wrongs that were done to him or her and the feelings those wrongs invoked, but also the wrongs he or she has done to his or her partner and the regrets those actions have caused.

In viewing both sides, the person will be able to overcome his or her bitterness and also his or her regret and learn from the lessons involved. The procedure for this Emotional First Aid subject, more than any other, requires a great balance between these two sides. If you haven't recently read the chapter titled Vital Information, do so now and then continue with the procedure that follows.

Compassion Remedy

The first step in handling a recent loss or trauma is to encourage the person to talk about it and to listen carefully to what the person says. Some encouragement may be needed at first. You can encourage a person to say more by use of the following prompts:

1. Tell me what happened.

2. Did anything else happen?

3. Is there anything else you want to tell me about that?

"When did you first realize there might be a (divorce) (separation) (abandonment) in the future?" is also a useful prompt. At no time during the conversation should you become critical or judgmental. Make a point of always letting the person know that you have heard what he or she is saying. A simple "uh huh" or "ok" is enough to acknowledge that you have heard someone. Most people will be very eager to talk to you as long as you remain compassionate and interested. You encourage the person to communicate fully by avoiding judgmental or critical communication or attitudes and by following the Golden Rules of Emotional First Aid. The person's recounting of the event may run for a few minutes or several hours. Be prepared to listen patiently throughout. If the person has told you about the incident but still has attention on it, ask him or her to tell you about it again one or more times.

Frequently, after telling you about the event, the person feels relieved and has no further interest in the event. If that is the case, end the Compassion Remedy at that point. If that is not the case, ask the person if there is something he or she now feels could be done about the event or if he or she now sees some way to handle the effects of the event in a positive manner. Looking at this point of view may help the person feel able to act as cause in the event rather than feeling victimized by it.

Check also for any decisions the person might have made at the time of the incident. Often a person makes major decisions during a time of loss and it is beneficial to take note of those decisions and to talk about them to a friend. Sometimes the decisions were wise ones and the talk reinforces them, but there are other times when the decisions would have proved to be destructive. An example might be someone who decides never to risk loving again because the loss was so painful. If left unexamined, that decision could prove to be harmful. Once the person has had the chance to talk about the loss at length and to begin the healing process, he or she might change his or her mind about the wisdom of such a decision. The spotting of decisions and communication about them with a compassionate listener is one of the most beneficial parts of this procedure. There may be one decision or many. Take plenty of time on this question and give the person the chance to examine all decisions.

If, during the course of doing this procedure, the person starts to speak of an earlier similar divorce, separation, or abandonment, go ahead and ask the person to examine that earlier time and ask the same series of questions about that incident.

When all decisions made at that earliest time have been viewed, the person will feel relieved and more extroverted and it is then time to end the procedure.

In the rare event that the person doesn't want to talk about the end of the relationship, encourage him or her to talk about the relationship itself, and when the person becomes more comfortable talking to you, he or she will quite naturally begin to speak of the end of the relationship.

It can take some time for the process of grieving to come to a closure.

If you feel the reactions of your friend or loved one to the incident are extreme, use the list of resources at the end of this section to encourage professional help. For the person who has strong ties to a religious group, there is often pastoral counseling available. For those who don't, many wonderful counseling centers exist where help can be obtained. The end of this section of the book contains references to help find professional help.

The Death of a Spouse

The death of a spouse is one of the most devastating losses a person will ever have to bear. The reaction to the loss may come immediately but more often comes later, after the initial dazed feeling lifts. Mourning is an important part of recovery as is the expression of grief.

The first step in helping the bereaved person may be very practical. The National Mental Health Association, in their pamphlet "Coping with Bereavement" recommends giving the following solid practical help:

"Offer to take care of children or cook an occasional meal. Invite them to your home. Such simple gestures can have priceless value to a family in shock."

Their next advice is to offer a listening ear. The simple procedure below offers a specific format to use to provide that compassionate listening ear. If you have not already done so, read the chapter called **Vital Information** before attempting to use the **Compassion Remedy.**

It is important to recognize that your goal in helping the person is not to have the person instantly recover completely and become to-

> ### Example
>
> *Kathy's husband had been sick for three years before his death. During that time, he had often suffered terrible pain. Kathy felt relief as well as grief when he finally died. She also felt guilty about having that sense of relief. When she received help for the loss, it was important for her to spot not only the moment when she first realized her husband would not survive his illness, but also to talk about her feelings of guilt. Kathy had time to say goodbye to her husband but needed to deal with her inability to help him survive.*
>
> *When Bill's wife died suddenly of a heart attack, his primary emotion was shock. In the course of helping him, it was important to focus heavily on the moment when he first received the shocking news, as well as on his subsequent feeling of being overwhelmed with grief. Bill also needed to talk about the fact that he had been unable to say goodbye.*

tally happy. That is an unrealistic goal. What you can do is help the person move freely and more rapidly through the stages of grief on their way to a full recovery. Sadly, it is not uncommon for a person to get hung up in one of the stages and spend years suffering because of it. Someone who receives help from a compassionate listener will recover from the feeling of terrible loss much more rapidly than someone who does not receive such help.

Keep in mind also that a spouse who has suffered a quick and unexpected loss is right at the beginning stage of recovery while a spouse who has had to deal with a long illness before the death may already have progressed through some of the stages of grief and so each may react differently. When the death follows a long illness, it is important to watch for the first point in time where the person realized his or her spouse might die as that point constitutes the beginning of the incident.

Compassion Remedy

The first step in handling a recent loss or trauma is to encourage the person to talk about it and to listen carefully to what the person says. Some encouragement may be needed at first. You can encourage a person to say more by use of the following prompts:

1. Tell me what happened.

2. Did anything else happen?

3. Is there anything else you want to tell me about that?

At no time during the conversation should you become critical or judgmental. Make a point of always letting the person know that you have heard what he or she is saying. A simple "uh huh" or "ok" is enough to acknowledge that you have heard someone. Most people will be very eager to talk to you as long as you remain compassionate and interested. You encourage the person to communicate fully by avoiding judgmental or critical communication or attitudes and by following the Golden Rules of Emotional First Aid. The person's recounting of the event may run for a few minutes or several hours. Be prepared to listen patiently throughout. If the person has told you about the incident but still has attention on it, ask him or her to tell you about it again one or more times.

Frequently, after telling you about the event, the person feels relieved and has no further interest in the event. If that is the case, end the Compassion Remedy at that point. If that is not the case, ask the person if there is something he or she now feels could be done about the event or if he or she now sees some way to handle the effects of the event in a positive manner. Looking at this point of view may help the person feel able to act as cause in the event rather than feeling victimized by it.

Check also for any decisions the person might have made at the time of the incident. Often a person makes major decisions during a time of loss and it is beneficial to take note of those decisions and to talk about them to a friend. Sometimes the decisions were wise ones and the talk reinforces them, but there are other times when the decisions would have proved to be destructive. An example might be someone who decides never to risk loving again because the loss was so painful. If left unexamined, that decision could prove to be harmful. Once the person has had the chance to talk about the loss at length and to begin the healing process, he or she might change his or her mind about the wisdom of such a decision. The spotting of decisions and communication about them with a compassionate listener is one of the most beneficial parts of this procedure. There may be one decision or many. Take plenty of time on this question and give the person the chance to examine all decisions.

When all decisions made at that earliest time have been viewed, the person will feel relieved and more extroverted and it is then time to end the procedure.

It can take some time for the complete healing process to occur. If you feel the reactions of your friend or loved one to the incident are extreme, use the list of resources in the appendix to encourage professional help. For the person who has strong ties to a religious group, there is often pastoral counseling available. For those who don't, many wonderful counseling centers exist where help can be obtained. The appendix of this book contains references to help find professional help.

Loss of Relationship—Mental Illness/Substance Abuse

There is a particular type of pain associated with watching the mental and physical destruction that accompanies serious mental illness and substance abuse. It would be almost impossible to watch such deterioration without suffering a sense of loss and failure. Examples of this are many: the spouse who watches a loved one stricken with Alzheimer's become unrecognizable; the parent who sees a bright, confident, loving child lose his or her happiness, peace, and confidence to Schizophrenia or Depression; the spouse who watches a partner disappear into an alcoholic fog. It differs from many of the other types of loss mentioned in this manual in that such a loss may drag out over a period of many years. The key to such a loss often lies in the point in time when the person actually gives up hope for improvement and decides that the situation is hopeless.

In addition to a feeling of loss for the person and his or her companionship, there is also a loss of the potential fulfillment of dreams that involved the other person. Examples include a parent who had dreams of a child's happy,

Example:

Lee took great delight in her youngest daughter, Stephanie, who was a bright charming little girl with tremendous potential. When Stephanie was stricken with Schizophrenia, Lee's dreams for her future were replaced by the constant stress of trying to deal with a frustrating and serious illness. Although Lee knew analytically that Stephanie was not to blame for her illness, it was difficult not to feel angry and frustrated with her child at times.

Lee's loss was very complex. Because the illness had taken over slowly, there was no clear-cut beginning and because there is currently no cure for the illness, there is no real end in sight either.

With patience and a great deal of compassion, Lee was able to express her grief, fear, and frustration. The help she received enabled her to better care for her daughter and for herself.

Lee also used the techniques in Section Two and Three of this book to provide Stephanie with emotional support.

secure future or a spouse who had dreamed of spending a pleasant old age in the company of their partner.

The Compassion Remedy that follows is designed to pick up these many aspects of the loss and allow the person to communicate fully about his or her feelings on each of these aspects.

Compassion Remedy

The first step in handling a recent loss or trauma is to encourage the person to talk about it and to listen carefully to what the person says. Some encouragement may be needed at first. You can encourage a person to say more by use of the following prompts:

1. Tell me what happened.

2. Did anything else happen?

3. Is there anything else you want to tell me about that?

At no time during the conversation should you become critical or judgmental. Make a point of always letting the person know that you have heard what he or she is saying. A simple "uh huh" or "ok" is enough to acknowledge that you have heard someone. Most people will be very eager to talk to you as long as you remain compassionate and interested. You encourage the person to communicate fully by avoiding judgmental or critical communication or attitudes and by following the Golden Rules of Emotional First Aid. The person's recounting of the event may run for a few minutes or several hours. Be prepared to listen patiently throughout. If the person has told you about the incident but still has attention on it, ask him or her to tell you about it again one or more times.

Frequently, after telling you about the event, the person feels relieved and has no further interest in the event. If that is the case, end the Compassion Remedy at that point. If that is not the case, ask the person if there is something he or she now feels could be done about the event or if he or she now sees some way to handle the effects of the event in a positive manner. Looking at this point of view may help the person feel able to act as cause in the event rather than feeling victimized by it.

Check also for any decisions the person might have made at the time of the incident. Often a person makes major decisions during a time of loss and it is beneficial to take note of those decisions and to talk about them to a friend. Sometimes the decisions were wise ones and the talk reinforces them, but there are other times when the decisions would have proved to be destructive. An example might be someone who decides not to get too close to others so he or she will never be hurt again. If left unexamined, that decision could prove to be harmful. Once the person has had the chance to talk about the loss at length and to begin the healing process, he or she might change his or her mind about the wisdom of such a decision. The spotting of decisions and communication about them with a compassionate listener is one of the most beneficial parts of this procedure. There may be one decision or many. Take plenty of time on this question and give the person the chance to examine all decisions.

If, during the course of doing this procedure, the person starts to speak of an earlier similar time when he or she felt a loss over watching someone deteriorate, go ahead and address that earlier time and ask the same series of questions about that incident.

When all decisions made at that earliest time have been viewed, the person will feel relieved and more extroverted and it is then time to end the procedure.

When someone is dealing with a serious mental illness or substance abuse, it is important to get help for them first. Once they have been helped, it may also be useful to introduce them to the techniques in Section Two and Three of this book. These techniques will help someone deal with the person who has the mental illness or substance abuse problem.

If you feel the reactions of your friend or loved one to the incident are extreme, use the list of resources in the appendix to encourage professional help. For the person who has strong ties to a religious group, there is often pastoral counseling available. For those who don't, many wonderful counseling centers exist where help can be obtained. The appendix of the book contains a complete listing of resources for obtaining such professional help.

Trauma of Infidelity

Is there a more crushing trauma in the world than this one? At the time it is happening to them, most people don't think so. Only the death of a child or other loved one outranks it on our lists of devastating experiences. Infidelity attacks at the root of our self-esteem and confidence like no other betrayal. Only a few tremendously confident people seem to come through such an experience relatively unscathed.

What is the hardest part of helping someone who has just discovered the infidelity of a spouse? Resisting the impulse to sympathize or take sides. Why must you resist it? You need to offer genuine help, and sympathy and prejudice are not compatible with effective help.

As noted in the Introduction to this section, sympathy—as opposed to empathy—is a way of saying that things really are awful and the person has been truly victimized by what has happened. There is a place for sympathy, but that place is not in the hands of the helper. If you were badly injured in a car accident and required therapy to recover all your ability, would you want a therapist who sympathized with you or one who effectively got you back on your feet? Would you want one who spent your precious session time agreeing with you about how awful the drunk driver who hit you was or one who focused completely on helping you get well? The loved one who has just discovered the unfaithfulness of a spouse has usually been hurt as badly as the automobile accident victim and is just as much in need of effective help.

Although there are cases where infidelity is totally caused by the actions of one of the parties, there are often actions taken by both parties that made the relationship vulnerable to this betrayal. Therefore it is equally important to make the person comfortable speaking of actions he or she might have taken that contributed to the problem. This is not done in order to assign blame. There is nothing in this Emotional First Aid Manual that is based on blame, shame, or regret. But it is most helpful to address both the areas where one is a victim of the actions of others and the areas where one contributed to the situation. Only then can the needed lessons be learned that will help us avoid a similar problem in the future. The only thing worse than experiencing infidelity once is having it happen more than once because the lessons that help avoid it weren't learned. This is why it is often equally important to help the person who initiated the infidelity if he or she wishes to be helped. Committing infidelity damages most people's self esteem and causes them the grief of knowing they have hurt their partner. It is only very rare cases where this is not true.

The point where the infidelity was discovered may be preceded by a period where it was only suspected. It's important to include this period in the events looked

---

Example

When Mary found her husband was seeing a coworker and had formed an adulterous relationship, she felt devastated. How could she not have known? Although she and her husband made the decision to continue the marriage after some marriage counseling, she could not get over the feeling of having been betrayed and the fear of the situation reoccurring.

When she was helped by the Compassion Remedy, she was able to realize that her tendency to stop communicating when she disagreed was damaging and that there had been signs of danger to the marriage that she ignored.

While her husband continued to work on the issues that had caused him to betray her, she was also able to improve the way she handled disagreements and to recognize and get help for danger signs before they became so serious that a betrayal resulted. Because of this, the marriage was actually strengthened. Even if the marriage had not been salvaged however, this knowledge would have helped her to prevent similar problems in future relationships.

---

at in the procedure that follows. That period of suspicion can be as stressful as the period of knowledge. It's also common to find infidelity repeated throughout a marriage. Watch for signs of an earlier incident as you do the procedure that follows.

Compassion Remedy

The first step in handling a recent loss or trauma is to encourage the person to talk about it and to listen carefully to what the person says. Some encouragement may be needed at first. You can encourage a person to say more by use of the following prompts:

1. Tell me what happened.

2. Did anything else happen?

3. Is there anything else you want to tell me about that?

At no time during the conversation should you become critical or judgmental. Make a point of always letting the person know that you have heard what he or she is saying. A simple "uh huh" or "ok" is enough to acknowledge that you have heard someone. Most people will be very eager to talk to you as long as you remain compassionate and interested. You encourage the person to communicate fully by avoiding judgmental or critical communication or attitudes and by following the Golden Rules of Emotional First Aid. The person's recounting of the event may run for a few minutes or several hours. Be prepared to listen patiently throughout. If the person has told you about the incident but still has attention on it, ask him or her to tell you about it again one or more times.

Frequently, after telling you about the event, the person feels relieved and has no further interest in the event. If that is the case, end the Compassion Remedy at that point. If that is not the case, ask the person if there is something he or she now feels could be done about the event or if he or she now sees some way to handle the effects of the event in a positive manner. Looking at this point of view may help the person feel able to act as cause in the event rather than feeling victimized by it.

Check also for any decisions the person might have made at the time of the incident. Often a person makes major decisions during a time of loss and it is beneficial to take note of those decisions and to talk about them to a friend. Sometimes the decisions were wise ones and the talk reinforces them, but there are other times when the decisions would have proved to be destructive. An example might be someone who decides not to get too close to others so he or she will never be hurt again. If left unexamined, that decision could prove to be harmful. Once the person has had the chance to talk about the loss at length and to begin the healing process, he or she might change his or her mind about the wisdom of such a decision. The spotting of decisions and communication about them with a compassionate listener is one of the most beneficial parts of this procedure. There may be one decision or many. Take plenty of time on this question and give the person the chance to examine all decisions.

If, during the course of doing this procedure, the person starts to speak of an earlier similar incident, go ahead and address that earlier time and ask the same series of questions about that incident.

When all decisions made at that earliest time have been viewed, the person will feel relieved and more extroverted and it is then time to end the procedure.

If you feel the reactions of your friend or loved one to the incident are extreme, use the list of resources in the appendix to encourage professional help. For the person who has strong ties to a religious group, there is often pastoral counseling available. For those who don't, many wonderful counseling centers exist where help can be obtained. The appendix of the book contains references to help find professional help.

Loss of Integrity

It's a rare person who can admit to a loss of integrity easily, but we have all experienced this problem. Some examples of a loss of integrity include the following:

- Succumbing to the temptation to cheat on a spouse

- Violating a tenet of one's religious beliefs

- Betraying an organization or person to whom one feels an allegiance

- Lying when it becomes uncomfortable to tell the truth

- Agreeing to something out of fear rather than conviction

- Pretending to be something one is not

When you observe a loved one or friend suffering from a loss of integrity or when a friend or loved one tells you of such a loss, first acknowledge his or her honesty in admitting that a lapse has occurred and then consider how great a loss this can be. There are few things in life more important than our wholeness of spirit or integrity. A lapse can be very painful and extremely damaging to one's self-esteem.

Example

Martin found himself spending too much money and then trying to hide his actions from his wife. This was causing him great stress since the actions went against his own code of ethics. When a friend of his used the Compassion Remedy to help him, Martin discovered some surprising decisions he had made in the past.

As a small boy, Martin had overheard a favorite uncle bemoaning the fact that his wife had left him when he went bankrupt. Martin was very disturbed by the fact that his uncle felt his wife only left him because he was not able to buy things for her.

He made a decision at that time that women could be very cruel and that it was best never to let them know if you were short of funds or you might end up grief stricken as his uncle seemed to be.

Martin realized his wife was a very different person from the woman his aunt had been and that the old decision was causing him to hide his actions today. Once he had realized that fact, he was able to change his mind about it and be honest with his wife without fear that she would leave him.

If you decide to help this friend or loved one, you will have to be very certain you can communicate on this subject with him or her in a compassionate, non-judgmental way. Even the slightest hint of criticism can destroy your ability to help. The person is already very aware of what he or she has done wrong. The need is to be able to examine the situation without having to defend his or her actions. If a conversation can occur that allows such an examination, enormous gains can be made. We learn from our lapses in integrity as long as we aren't so busy defending our actions that we have no time to learn from them. Part of the procedure that follows involves having the person who lost his or her integrity examine the actions, thoughts, and feelings that led to such a lapse. In doing this examination, realizations will occur that will aid the person in not committing the error again. All the advice or admonishments in the world won't necessarily lead to a change, but this process of self-examination may do so.

If you haven't recently done so, reread the Chapter called Vital Information. You will need to have the Seven Golden Rules of Emotional First Aid clearly in mind to use the following procedure to help you friend or loved one.

Compassion Remedy

The first step in handling the loss of integrity is to let the person talk about when he or she first began to betray his or her own integrity and then look at the period just prior to that to identify what fear or trauma led him or her to do so. It's important for the person to look at both the trauma that led to the loss of integrity as well as the effects on his or her life of the loss. Some encouragement may be needed at first. You can encourage a person to say more by use of the following prompts:

1. Tell me what happened.

2. Did anything else happen?

3. Is there anything else you want to tell me about that?

At no time during the conversation should you become critical or judgmental. Make a point of always letting the person know that you have heard what he or she is saying. A simple "uh huh" or "ok" is enough to acknowledge that you have heard someone. Most people will be very eager to talk to you as long as you remain compassionate and interested. You encourage the person to communicate fully by avoiding judgmental or critical communication or attitudes and by following the Golden Rules of Emotional First Aid. The person's recounting of the event may run for a few minutes or several hours. Be prepared to listen patiently throughout. If the person has told you about the incident but still has attention on it, ask him or her to tell you about it again one or more times.

Frequently, after telling you about the event, the person feels relieved and has no further interest in the event. If that is the case, end the Compassion Remedy at that point. If that is not the case, ask the person if there is something he or she now feels could be done about the event or if he or she now sees some way to handle the effects of the event in a positive manner. Looking at this point of view may help the person feel able to act as cause in the event rather than feeling victimized by it.

Check also for any decisions the person might have made at the time of the incident. Often a person makes major decisions during a time of loss and it is beneficial to take note of those decisions and to talk about them to a friend. Sometimes the decisions were wise ones and the talk reinforces them, but there are other times when the decisions would have proved to be destructive. An example might be someone who decides never to trust himself or herself again. If left unexamined, that decision could prove to be harmful. Once the person has had the chance to talk about the loss at length and to begin the healing process, he or she might change his or her mind about the wisdom of such a decision. The spotting of decisions and communication about them with a compassionate listener is one of the most beneficial parts of this procedure. There may be one decision or many. Take plenty of time on this question and give the person the chance to examine all decisions.

If, during the course of doing this procedure, the person starts to speak of an earlier similar incident, go ahead and focus on that earlier time and ask the same series of questions about that incident.

When all decisions made at that earliest time have been viewed, the person will feel relieved and more extroverted and it is then time to end the procedure.

If you feel the reactions of your friend or loved one to the incident are extreme, use the list of resources in the appendix to encourage professional help. For the person who has strong ties to a religious group, there is often pastoral counseling available. For those who don't, many wonderful counseling centers exist where help can be obtained. The appendix contains references to help find professional help.

Trauma of False Accusations

As anyone knows, false accusations can be extremely painful. For many people there's an added source of pain since they lack the skills to be able to disprove such accusations. A false accusation, given enough power by the stature of the accuser can cause permanent damage to a vulnerable person. Without the ability to disprove the accusation, this person can be wrongly branded for life, a fact that not only influences how others treat him or her, but also how the person feels about himself or herself.

Certainly when you see a friend or loved one being falsely accused, it's necessary to take it seriously and do everything possible to help make the truth widely known. It's also helpful to allow the person to express fully the grief, outrage, and fear that can result from such accusations.

We've all heard the strength of someone's protest that, "It's not fair!" People have an innate sense of what is or isn't fair and they take violations of the "fairness" very hard. False accusations strike hard at that sense of fairness.

When an accusation is false, it may be that the person who is accused is completely blameless or simply that he or she did not do the action stated although another action was done that was destructive. Either way, the person is deserving of help. Make it very

Example

Mike was accused by his employer of stealing a tool from the workplace. This accusation was made in front of many of his friends and coworkers and caused his extreme embarrassment. The stress was severe enough that Mike was unable to sleep well because of his embarrassment and fear of losing his job.

In the course of doing the Compassion Remedy, Mike told the friend who was helping him that, while he had not stolen the tool, he had once taken home some items from work that he had been ordered to dispose of by his employer.

Mike's friend wisely continued the procedure and Mike experienced relief from the stress and an increased ability to handle the workplace incident.

Stopping the procedure because Mike had done something wrong in the past would have prevented him from making these gains.

safe for the person to tell you if he or she did do something that is now regretted. By showing compassion, you can make it possible for the person to admit any wrongdoing that did occur while still experiencing relief by speaking of what was false about the accusations. Rarely, you may start to help someone who says he or she was wrongly accused and then find the person admitting part way through the procedure that the accusation was actually correct. If so, continue the procedure anyway. It is very traumatic to have made a mistake and then have it advertised to the world. The person is still deserving of your help.

The procedure that follows is designed to allow you to help your friend or loved one to recover fully from this particular example of the unfairness of life.

Compassion Remedy

The first step in handling a recent loss or trauma is to encourage the person to talk about it and to listen carefully to what the person says. Some encouragement may be needed at first. You can encourage a person to say more by use of the following questions

1. Tell me what happened.

2. Did anything else happen?

3. Is there anything else you want to tell me about that?

At no time during the conversation should you become critical or judgmental. Make a point of always letting the person know that you have heard what he or she is saying. A simple "uh huh" or "ok" is enough to acknowledge that you have heard someone. Most people will be very eager to talk to you as long as you remain compassionate and interested. You encourage the person to communicate fully by avoiding judgmental or critical communication or attitudes and by following the Golden Rules of Emotional First Aid. The person's recounting of the event may run for a few minutes or several hours. Be prepared to listen patiently throughout. If the person has told you about the incident but still has attention on it, ask him or her to tell you about it again one or more times.

Frequently, after telling you about the event, the person feels relieved and has no further interest in the event. If that is the case, end the Compassion Remedy at that point. If that is not the case, ask the person if there is something he or she now feels could be done about the event or if he or she now sees some way to handle the effects of the event in a positive manner. Looking at this point of view may help the person feel able to act as cause in the event rather than feeling victimized by it.

Check also for any decisions the person might have made at the time of the incident. Often someone makes major decisions during a time of stress and it is beneficial to take note of those decisions and to talk about them to a friend or loved one. Sometimes the decisions were wise ones and the talk reinforces them, but there are other times when the decisions would have proved to be destruc- tive. An example might be a person who decides he or she is worth- less because of the accusations. If left unexamined, that decision could prove to be harmful. Once the person has had the chance to talk about the upset at length and to begin the healing process, he or she might change his or her mind about the wisdom of such a decision. The spotting of decisions and communication about them with a compassionate listener is one of the most beneficial parts of this procedure. There may be one decision or many. Take plenty of time on this question and give the person the chance to examine all decisions.

If, during the course of doing this procedure, the person starts to speak of an earlier similar upset, go ahead and focus on that earlier time and ask the same series of questions about that incident.

When all decisions made at that earliest time have been viewed, the person will feel relieved and more extroverted and it is then time to end the procedure.

If you feel the reactions of your friend or loved one to the incident are extreme, use the list of resources in the appendix to encourage professional help. For the person who has strong ties to a religious group, there is often pastoral counseling available. For those who don't, many wonderful counseling centers exist where help can be obtained. The appendix of the book contains references to help find professional help.

Loss of Recreational Time

This topic might be taken more lightly than others in this book by someone who hasn't considered it carefully but a loss of recreational time can involve serious emotional stress. When financial problems, single parenthood, family responsibilities, caretaking duties, or other hardships cause someone to lose out on any recreational time, it can ultimately cause damage to that person's health as well as emotional burnout.

There are "in life" ways to help a friend or loved one who has no recreational time. An offer to a person whose spouse has Alzheimer's, for example, to care for his or her spouse for a few hours a week while the caregiver attends an Alzheimer's Support Group is a possibility. There, the friend or loved one will find people who can help him or her locate additional support and relief.

An offer to a friend who is struggling as a single parent to take his or her children on an outing while the friend also checks out groups like Parents without Partners might be another way to help. Anyone who is overburdened with responsibility can use a few free hours a week.

Example:

Mary's father suffers from Alzheimer's disease and Mary has taken over his full-time care. Because her father must be watched closely at all times, and because financial hardships prevent her from being able to hire help that might give her relief, Mary has given up all her former recreational pursuits. Her father may live for many years yet and Mary has begun to see her life as a long unending cycle of responsibility and drudgery.

Help given to Mary through the Compassion Remedy in this manual may enable her to be more assertive in finding support through the organizations who provide it.

Example:

Tom is a single parent with three children to support. His wages as a schoolteacher barely cover the cost of living and child care. Tom's youngest child has medical problems that create additional financial hardship.

Tom is exhausted frequently and spends his little free time caring for the children's needs and trying to substitute emotionally for their missing mother. He sees long years ahead with no easing of responsibility or return of free time for his own needs.

With help, Tom may begin to reach out for some of the support available.

In addition to this practical help is the help that can be given by a compassionate listener. The procedure that follows is something else you can do to offer help to such a friend.

Compassion Remedy

The first step in handling a recent loss of recreational time is to encourage the person to talk about it and to listen carefully to what the person says. Some encouragement may be needed at first. You can encourage a person to say more by use of the following questions

1. Tell me what happened.

2. Did anything else happen?

3. Is there anything else you want to tell me about that?

At no time during the conversation should you become critical or judgmental. Make a point of always letting the person know that you have heard what he or she is saying. A simple "uh huh" or "ok" is enough to acknowledge that you have heard someone. Most people will be very eager to talk to you as long as you remain compassionate and interested. You encourage the person to communicate fully by avoiding judgmental or critical communication or attitudes and by following the Golden Rules of Emotional First Aid. The person's recounting of the event may run for a few minutes or several hours. Be prepared to listen patiently throughout. If the person has told you about the incident but still has attention on it, ask him or her to tell you about it again one or more times.

Frequently, after telling you about the event, the person feels relieved and has no further interest in the event. If that is the case, end the Compassion Remedy at that point. If that is not the case, ask the person if there is something he or she now feels could be done about the event or if he or she now sees some way to handle the effects of the event in a positive manner. Looking at this point of view may help the person feel able to act as cause in the event rather than feeling victimized by it.

Check also for any decisions the person might have made at the time of the incident. Often someone makes major decisions during a time of stress and it is beneficial to take note of those decisions and to talk about them to a friend or loved one. Sometimes the decisions were wise ones and the talk reinforces them, but there are other times when the decisions would have proved to be destructive. An example might be a person who decides he or she might as well give up on trying to have a life. If left unexamined, that decision could prove to be harmful. Once the person has had the chance to talk about the upset at length and to begin the healing process, he or she might change his or her mind about the wisdom of such a decision. The spotting of decisions and communication about them with a compassionate listener is one of the most beneficial parts of this procedure. There may be one decision or many. Take plenty of time on this question and give the person the chance to examine all decisions.

If, during the course of doing this procedure, the person starts to speak of an earlier similar upset, go ahead and focus on that earlier time and ask the same series of questions about that incident.

When all decisions made at that earliest time have been viewed, the person will feel relieved and more extroverted and it is then time to end the procedure.

If you feel the emotional reactions of your friend or loved one are extreme, use the list of resources in the appendix to find professional help. For the family that has strong ties to a religious group, there is often pastoral counseling available. For those who don't, many wonderful counseling centers exist where help can be obtained. The appendix of the book contains resources for obtaining such professional help.

Trauma Due to a Legal Situation

The majority of the population (with the obvious exception of attorneys) find legal threats among the most traumatic situations in the world. The thought of a trip to court stimulates memories of childhood trips to the principal's office, punishment by parents and teachers, and other unpleasant brushes with authority. In addition, the high cost of legal protection adds the picture of financial damage or ruin to the situation for most people.

A friend or loved one undergoing any type of legal action is likely to be feeling tremendous emotional stress. This stress affects not only the actual participant in the legal action, but also the family members who endure it with him or her.

> *Example:*
>
> *John had invested in a business that is now being sued by a major client. Although he had only limited interaction with this business and none with the client, his financial future is now at risk along with the active participants. John is 60 years old and it is his retirement money at stake. The stress of worrying about his own future, as well as that of his wife, is keeping him awake night after night and is aggravating his high blood pressure.*
>
> *Some help from the Compassion Remedy might enable him to stay calm enough to sleep well so he can plan his legal strategy and keep his health at the same time.*

All the people in these examples could use help from their friends and loved ones, but embarrassment over the circumstances may make it hard for them to speak freely to someone who wants to help. In this type of situation, your ability to be a very compassionate, completely non-judgmental listener is vital. One hint of a critical attitude or word will bar you from being able to relieve the suffering. Keep clearly in mind that whether or not the person or his or her loved one is guilty or innocent as far as the legal arena is concerned is irrelevant to the fact that he or she is suffering.

It is the court's job to determine right or wrong and to handle any punishment. Your job, if you choose to try to help this friend or loved one, is to listen compassionately to his or her fears, hopes, and considerations. A person who has made a mistake is better able to change the destructive behavior if there is at least one person he or she can talk to without feeling the need to defend his or her actions. Use the Compassion Remedy below to provide that opportunity for your friends or loved ones to unburden themselves.

Compassion Remedy

The first step in handling the emotional stress of a legal threat is to encourage the person to talk about it and to listen carefully to what the person says. Some encouragement may be needed at first. You can encourage a person to say more by use of the following questions

> *Example:*
>
> *Alice and Mike's 19-year-old son, Frank, is accused of cheating on a test at the Military Academy. Although the most severe penalty threatened is expulsion from the Academy, Frank's parents see their son's whole career and self esteem at stake. They are terribly disturbed at this threat to the son they dearly love.*
>
> *The result of help from the Compassion Remedy will make it possible for them to do what is best for their son and also to help their son talk about his feelings to them without fear of upsetting them further.*

1. Tell me what happened.

2. Did anything else happen?

3. Is there anything else you want to tell me about that?

At no time during the conversation should you become critical or judgmental. Make a point of always letting the person know that you have heard what he or she is saying. A simple "uh huh" or "ok" is enough to acknowledge that you have heard someone. Most people will be very eager to talk to you as long as you remain compassionate and interested. You encourage the person to communicate fully by avoiding judgmental or critical communication or attitudes and by following the Golden Rules of Emotional First Aid. The person's recounting of the event may run for a few minutes or several hours. Be prepared to listen patiently throughout. If the person has told you about the incident but still has attention on it, ask him or her to tell you about it again one or more times.

Frequently, after telling you about the event, the person feels relieved and has no further interest in the event. If that is the case, end the Compassion Remedy at that point. If that is not the case, ask the person if there is something he or she now feels could be done about the event or if he or she now sees some way to handle the effects of the event in a positive manner. Looking at this point of view may help the person feel able to act as cause in the event rather than feeling victimized by it.

Check also for any decisions the person might have made at the time of the incident. Often someone makes major decisions during a time of stress and it is beneficial to take note of those decisions and to talk about them to a friend or loved one. Sometimes the decisions were wise ones and the talk reinforces them, but there are other times when the decisions would have proved to be destructive. An example might be a person who decides the situation is hopeless. If left unexamined, that decision could prove to be harmful. Once the person has had the chance to talk about the upset at length and to begin the healing process, he or she might change his or her mind about the wisdom of such a decision. The spotting of decisions and communication about them with a compassionate listener is one of the most beneficial parts of this procedure. There may be one decision or many. Take plenty of time on this question and give the person the chance to examine all decisions.

If, during the course of doing this procedure, the person starts to speak of an earlier similar upset, go ahead and focus on that earlier time and ask the same series of questions about that incident.

When all decisions made at that earliest time have been viewed, the person will feel relieved and more extroverted and it is then time to end the procedure.

If you feel the emotional reactions of your friend or loved one are extreme, use the list of resources in the appendix to find professional help. For the family that has strong ties to a religious group, there is often pastoral counseling available. For those who don't, many wonderful counseling centers exist where help can be obtained. The appendix at the end of the book contains resources for obtaining such professional help.

Trauma of Betrayal

Betrayal — Even the word gives most people the chills. And it doesn't matter if the betrayal is real or the result of a misperception or misunderstanding. The devastation and desolation caused by feeling betrayed is overpowering. This is one of those emotions that goes right to the core of our feelings about our worth and our self-esteem.

Feelings of betrayal may set the stage for a person's life-long attitudes about his or her fellow human beings. Don't ever underestimate the power of this emotion and do provide all the help you can for a friend or loved one who is suffering from this feeling. The procedure below will help you provide that aid.

Example:

When there was a management change at the company where Susan worked, she thought the rewards of her many years of outstanding production would carry over. They didn't. In short order, the new management had replaced her with their own candidate for the job and Susan found herself out in the cold. The sense of betrayal she felt colored her whole feeling toward life and she found it almost impossible to gain the confidence she needed to begin a successful job search.

A friend who helped her communicate about her feelings enabled her to move on and continue the job search with enough confidence to get a new job that was rewarding.

Compassion Remedy

The first step in handling the trauma of betrayal is to encourage the person to talk about it and to listen carefully to what the person says. Some encouragement may be needed at first. You can encourage a person to say more by use of the following questions

1. Tell me what happened.

2. Did anything else happen?

3. Is there anything else you want to tell me about that?

At no time during the conversation should you become critical or judgmental. Make a point of always letting the person know that you have heard what he or she is saying. A simple "uh huh" or "ok" is enough to acknowledge that you have heard someone. Most people will be very eager to talk to you as long as you remain compassionate and interested. You encourage the person to communicate fully by avoiding judgmental or critical communication or attitudes and by following the Golden Rules of Emotional First Aid. The person's recounting of the event may run for a few minutes or several hours. Be prepared to listen patiently throughout. If the person has told you about the incident but still has attention on it, ask him or her to tell you about it again one or more times.

> **Example**
>
> *When Henry told his closest friend in confidence of the failure of his business, he never expected his wounded feelings and confessions of inadequacy would become the subject of casual conversation. When a mutual acquaintance alluded to this painful subject in a manner that showed his knowledge of the personal details, Henry felt betrayed by his friend. His anger spelled the end of a long and otherwise rewarding friendship.*
>
> *As noted in the chapter of this book called Vital Information, it is critical to respect the privacy of others when you are using the procedures in this book. If you fail to do so, you will have created a new trauma rather than relieving an old one.*

Frequently, after telling you about the event, the person feels relieved and has no further interest in the event. If that is the case, end the Compassion Remedy at that point. If that is not the case, ask the person if there is something he or she now feels could be done about the event or if he or she now sees some way to handle the effects of the event in a positive manner. Looking at this point of view may help the person feel able to act as cause in the event rather than feeling victimized by it.

Check also for any decisions the person might have made at the time of the incident. Often someone makes major decisions during a time of stress and it is beneficial to take note of those decisions and to talk about them to a friend or parent. Sometimes the decisions were wise ones and the talk reinforces them, but there are other times when the decisions would have proved to be destructive. An example might be a person who decides never to trust someone again because the potential for betrayal is too great. If left unexamined, that decision could prove to be harmful. Once the person has had the chance to talk about the loss at length and to begin the healing process, he or she might change his or her mind about the wisdom of such a decision. The spotting of decisions and communication about them with a compassionate listener is one of the most beneficial parts of this procedure. There may be one decision or many. Take plenty of time on this question and give the person the chance to examine all decisions.

If, during the course of doing this procedure, the person starts to speak of an earlier similar loss, go ahead and focus on that earlier time and ask the same series of questions about that incident.

When all decisions made at that earliest time have been viewed, the person will feel relieved and more extroverted and it is then time to end the procedure.

If you feel the emotional reactions of your friend or loved one are extreme, use the list of resources at the end of this section to find professional help. For the family that has strong ties to a religious group, there is often pastoral counseling available. For those who don't, many wonderful counseling centers exist where help can be obtained. The end of this section of the book contains information on resources for obtaining such professional help.

Loss of Reputation

Is there a person on this planet with a strong enough sense of self-esteem to withstand damage to—or the loss of—his or her reputation without severe emotional stress? Is it less painful if the loss was deserved?

No! That's the answer to both of the questions above.

Whether we're an innocent victim of circumstances or we lost our reputation through our own mistakes, the resulting stress and trauma is often more than our delicate sense of self-esteem can handle and we almost always suffer lifelong damage without proper and effective help. The fact that we may have made mistakes that led to the loss doesn't mean we shouldn't receive any help in relieving the stress caused by the loss. Severe stress can ruin our health and make us less able to make amends for whatever mistakes have been made. Even if we are angry about the destructiveness of the events that led to the loss of the reputation, it is still in our best interests to try to help the person involved. When people are helped in a truly compassionate way, they are more likely to change the destructive behavior that led to the loss of reputation than if others just want them to suffer.

Example:

Mark was arrested one day for embezzlement and the news of his situation was trumpeted in the local newspapers and news broadcasts. The resulting legal actions dragged out for two years and the story was replaced in the headlines by newer, more newsworthy stories. When he was finally cleared of all charges, it was a minor footnote on the back page. Mark's professional and personal reputation suffered greatly from the negative publicity. But the damage to his career paled in comparison to the damage to his sense of well being and self-esteem. Without help, it could honestly be said that Mark would never fully recover from his bitterness and grief.

Fortunately a good friend was able to provide the needed help and Mark rebuilt his career and his happiness.

The procedure used to help a friend or loved one who has lost his or her reputation is identical whether the loss was deserved or not.

Both situations require the most compassionate and non-judgmental hearing possible. This procedure is designed to help you offer your friends and loved ones that level of kindness and effective help.

Compassion Remedy

The first step in handling the emotional trauma of a loss of reputation is to let the person talk about when he or she first began to realize that his or her reputation had been damaged and to listen carefully to what the person says. Some encouragement may be needed at first. You can encourage a person to say more by use of the following prompts:

1. Tell me what happened.

2. Did anything else happen?

3. Is there anything else you want to tell me about that?

At no time during the conversation should you become critical or judgmental. Make

> *Example:*
>
> *Carol, a survivor of a childhood marred by physical and sexual abuse, went through four marriages and messy divorces before she finally began to get the help needed to enable her to have a stable and successful relationship. By the time she got that help, her reputation as a wife and mother in the small town where she lived had suffered heavily from the years of failure in her relationships. Carol felt overwhelmed by the job of trying to live down that reputation. She eventually moved to a larger city, leaving behind friends and family, just to avoid being confronted by the gossip that had circled around her.*
>
> *Even in the new location, however, she would benefit from being able to handle the stress of her lost reputation. Otherwise, she will live in fear of bumping into an old acquaintance from her hometown.*

a point of always letting the person know that you have heard what he or she is saying. A simple "uh huh" or "ok" is enough to acknowledge that you have heard someone. Most people will be very eager to talk to you as long as you remain compassionate and interested. You encourage the person to communicate fully by avoiding judgmental or critical communication or attitudes and by following the Golden Rules of Emotional First Aid. The person's recounting of the event may run for a few minutes or several hours. Be prepared to listen patiently throughout. If the person has told you about the incident but still has attention on it, ask him or her to tell you about it again one or more times.

Frequently, after telling you about the event, the person feels relieved and has no further interest in the event. If that is the case, end the Compassion Remedy at that point. If that is not the case, ask the person if there is something he or she now feels could be done about the event or if he or she now sees some way to handle the effects of the event in a positive manner. Looking at this point of view may help the person feel able to act as cause in the event rather than feeling victimized by it.

Check also for any decisions the person might have made at the time of the incident. Often someone makes major decisions during a time of stress and it is beneficial to take note of those decisions and to talk about them to a friend or loved one. Sometimes the decisions were wise ones and the talk reinforces them, but there are other times when the decisions would have proved to be destructive. An example might be a person who decides he or she is worthless because of the loss. If left unexamined, that decision could prove to be harmful. Once the person has had the chance to talk about the upset at length and to begin the healing process, he or she might change his or her mind about the wisdom of such a decision. The spotting of decisions and communication about them with a compassionate listener is one of the most beneficial parts of this procedure. There may be one decision or many. Take plenty of time on this question and give the person the chance to examine all decisions.

If, during the course of doing this procedure, the person starts to speak of an earlier similar upset, go ahead and focus on that earlier time and ask the same series of questions about that incident.

When all decisions made at that earliest time have been viewed, the person will feel relieved and more extroverted and it is then time to end the procedure.

If you feel the emotional reactions of your friend or loved one are extreme, use the list of resources in the appendix to find professional help. For the family that has strong ties to a religious group, there is often pastoral counseling available. For those who don't, many wonderful counseling centers exist where help can be obtained. The appendix of the book contains resources for obtaining such professional help.

Loss of a Child, Infant, or Fetus

There are very few people in the world who would not agree that the loss of a child is the single most painful loss anyone could ever experience. The fierce protective drive that nature has built into parents to ensure the survival of our species, coupled with the incredible love of most parents for their children, as well as the feeling of unfairness when a young life is cut short are all overwhelming factors in that grief.

Most of us find ourselves frightened in the face of such pain, wondering what we can possibly say or do that would offer comfort to the grieving family. It's very important for us to remember that it isn't what we say that is important; there are no words that can offer much comfort to a family that has lost a child. It is our ability to be a compassionate listener that will offer real help. In addition to grief, family members are also

Example:

Wendy lost her son to Sudden Infant Death Syndrome when the child was less than six months old. She was inconsolable. Her sister, Janice, was close to her and Janice tried to bring Wendy out of her shell. Janice was able to be of some help by getting Wendy to open up and finally talk about the loss. One day, however, Wendy, encouraged by the fact that Janice had been so willing to listen, dared to express how angry she felt at God for not preventing the death. Janice, who was a strongly religious person, felt her God was being attacked by Wendy's comments and she began to try to talk Wendy out of the idea that it was God's fault.

Wendy immediately sensed that her anger was unacceptable and upsetting to Janice and, because she loved her sister and did not want to hurt her, she stopped expressing her anger though she still felt it. Janice's ability to help Wendy came to an end at that point as Wendy no longer viewed her as a safe person to talk to on that subject. Wendy was unable to overcome her grief for many years and never dared during that time to chance having another child. Finally, five years later, a perceptive minister, in the course of checking into why Wendy's participation in her own church had dropped off, was able to get Wendy to open up once again. He wisely let Wendy express her anger fully. Wendy began to progress in her recovery at that point and today has had another child as well as a re-establishment of her relationship with God and with her church.

suffering from many less "acceptable" emotions. Anger is the most prominent among these; anger at a God who allowed this to happen, anger at the medical staff that couldn't prevent the death, anger at themselves for somehow being responsible. It is vital to the mourners to be able to vent all their emotions, even those strong feelings of anger, resentment, bitterness, guilt, and injustice, and the person listening to them must be compassionate and must refrain from trying to talk them out of those feelings.

It often takes months or years to pass through the acute stages of grief. Don't expect an instant recovery when you use the procedures in this book to help. If you apply them well, however, you can contribute to that acute stage taking only weeks or months rather than years, and that is a major contribution.

The resource list in the appendix contains the names of some excellent support groups for grieving families. You can send for material from them to pass along to your friend or loved one and we strongly recommend that you do so. These support groups are excellent sources of help. We also strongly recommend that you encourage your loved one to get some professional help. The organizations noted often can give you names of professionals in your area who specialize in working with grieving families.

Don't underestimate the help you can give to your friends and loved ones using the procedures that follow. It takes a lot of courage to step in and invite that loved one to communicate about his or her pain, but if you follow through, it will be one of the most rewarding things you've ever done.

Calming Procedure

As noted in the introduction to this section, there are actions that can be taken in life to help someone who has lost a child. Do as many of these actions as it is possible for you to do.

- ❐ Help create a calm, quiet, predictable environment for the traumatized person

- ❐ Encourage the person to get extra nutritional support (stress burns more nutrients)

❏ Treat the person as gently as possible recognizing that an emotional injury is as destructive as a physical one

❏ Give as much physical contact as appropriate and acceptable: hugs, hand holding, pats on the shoulder, etc.

❏ Be reassuring whenever possible but don't attempt to make less of the loss or try to talk the person out of his or her feelings

❏ Help provide the presence of a compassionate adult until the worst of the trauma has passed

❏ Provide as much unconditional love as you can

Compassion Remedy

The best way to contribute to helping with the emotional trauma of losing a child is to encourage the person talk about when he or she first began to realize that a loss was imminent or that, in the case of a sudden death, a loss had occurred. Some encouragement may be needed at first. You can encourage a person to say more by use of the following prompts:

1. Tell me what happened.

2. Did anything else happen?

3. Is there anything else you want to tell me about that?

At no time during the conversation should you become critical or judgmental. Make a point of always letting the person know that you have heard what he or she is saying. A simple "uh huh" or "ok" is enough to acknowledge that you have heard someone. Most people will be very eager to talk to you as long as you remain compassionate and interested. You encourage the person to communicate fully by avoiding judgmental or critical communication or attitudes and by following the Golden Rules of Emotional First Aid. The person's recounting of the event may run for a few minutes or several hours. Be prepared to listen patiently throughout. If the person has told you about the incident but still has attention on it, ask him or her to tell you about it again one or more times.

Frequently, after telling you about the event, the person feels relieved and has no further interest in the event. If that is the case, end the Compassion Remedy at that point. If that is not the case, ask the person if there is something he or she now feels could be done about the event or if he or she now sees some way to handle the effects of the event in a positive manner. Looking at this point of view may help the person feel able to act as cause in the event rather than feeling victimized by it.

Check also for any decisions the person might have made at the time of the incident. Often someone makes major decisions during a time of stress and it is beneficial to take note of those decisions and to talk about them to a friend or loved one. Sometimes the decisions were wise ones and the talk reinforces them, but there are other times when the decisions would have proved to be destructive. An example might be a person who decides that he or she is not a good parent because of the loss. If left unexamined, that decision could prove to be harmful. Once the person has had the chance to talk about the upset at length and to begin the healing process, he or she might change his or her mind about the wisdom of such a decision. The spotting of decisions and communication about them with a compassionate listener is one of the most beneficial parts of this procedure. There may be one decision or many. Take plenty of time on this question and give the person the chance to examine all decisions.

If, during the course of doing this procedure, the person starts to speak of an earlier similar upset, go ahead and focus on that earlier time and ask the same series of questions about that incident.

When all decisions made at that earliest time have been viewed, the person will feel relieved and more extroverted and it is then time to end the procedure.

In the case of the loss of a child, it is best to use the list of resources in the appendix to find professional help in addition to the emotional first aid you can provide. For the family that has strong ties to a religious group, there is often pastoral counseling available. For those who don't, many wonderful counseling centers exist where help can be obtained. The appendix of the book contains resources for obtaining such professional help.

Loss of Parent, Grandparent, or Family Member

It is inevitable, as you go through life, that you will have a friend or a loved one who suffers the loss of a close family member. Although many of us feel awkward about knowing what to say at those times, it's important to remember that we are not required to say profoundly comforting things. It is our ability to listen compassionately that we can offer as a gift to our loved ones, not our ability to know just the right thing to say. This knowledge comes as a relief to most of us as it is far easier to encourage a person to talk about a loss than it is to come up with words of wisdom that will help heal them.

Calming Procedure

As noted in the introduction to this section, there are actions that can be taken in life to help someone who has lost a loved one. Do as many of these actions as it is possible for you to do.

❒ Help create a calm, quiet, predictable environment for the traumatized person

❒ Encourage the person to get extra nutritional support (stress burns more nutrients)

❒ Treat the person as gently as possible recognizing that an emotional injury is as destructive as a physical one

❒ Give as much physical contact as appropriate and acceptable: hugs, hand holding, pats on the shoulder, etc.

❒ Be reassuring whenever possible but don't attempt to make less of the loss or try to talk the person out of his or her feelings

❒ Help provide the presence of a compassionate adult until the worst of the trauma has passed

❒ Provide as much unconditional love as you can

Then read the procedure that follows and give it a try with your loved one. As long as you follow the Golden Rules of Emotional First Aid, you can't cause any harm and you may be able to provide a great deal of help.

Compassion Remedy

The first step in handling the emotional trauma of losing a close family member is to let the person talk about when he or she first began to realize that a loss was imminent or, in the case of a sudden death, when he or she first heard about or saw the death occur. Some encouragement may be needed at first. You can encourage a person to say more by use of the following prompts:

1. Tell me what happened.

2. Did anything else happen?

3. Is there anything else you want to tell me about that?

At no time during the conversation should you become critical or judgmental. Make a point of always letting the person know that you have heard what he or she is saying. A simple "uh huh" or "ok" is enough to acknowledge that you have heard someone. Most people will be very eager to talk to you as

> **Example**
>
> *When John lost his father, it was a complex loss. Not only did he miss the man who had reared him, he became the patriarch of his family, a role he didn't feel prepared to fill. John also had some complex feelings toward his father. While his father was a good man, he was not easy to please. John was never sure he had made his father proud and now he felt he had lost the opportunity to do so. Like most of us, John had very mixed feelings about the death and some of them were difficult to express.*
>
> *When John was helped by a particularly compassionate friend, he was able to look at and discuss his father for the first time as an adult. In the course of doing the Compassion Remedy in this book he discovered he had made some important decisions in the past. He had decided he could never be the equal of his father, that he could never please him, and that he was a poor father himself. Those decisions were obscured by his strong emotions until he had spoken of his loss at length. Finally he was able to re-examine the decisions and the circumstances under which they were made and change his mind about their validity.*

long as you remain compassionate and interested. You encourage the person to communicate fully by avoiding judgmental or critical communication or attitudes and by following the Golden Rules of Emotional First Aid. The person's recounting of the event may run for a few minutes or several hours. Be prepared to listen patiently throughout. If the person has told you about the incident but still has attention on it, ask him or her to tell you about it again one or more times.

Frequently, after telling you about the event, the person feels relieved and has no further interest in the event. If that is the case, end the Compassion Remedy at that point. If that is not the case, ask the person if there is something he or she now feels could be done about the event or if he or she now sees some way to handle the effects of the event in a positive manner. Looking at this point of view may help the person feel able to act as cause in the event rather than feeling victimized by it.

Check also for any decisions the person might have made at the time of the incident. Often someone makes major decisions during a time of stress and it is beneficial to take note of those decisions and to talk about them to a friend or loved one. Sometimes the decisions were wise ones and the talk reinforces them, but there are other times when the decisions would have proved to be destructive. An example might be a person who decides not to get too close to others so that their eventual loss is not as painful. If left unexamined, that decision could prove to be harmful. Once the person has had the chance to talk about the upset at length and to begin the healing process, he or she might change his or her mind about the wisdom of such a decision. The spotting of decisions and communication about them with a compassionate listener is one of the most beneficial parts of this procedure. There may be one decision or many. Take plenty of time on this question and give the person the chance to examine all decisions.

If, during the course of doing this procedure, the person starts to speak of an earlier similar upset, go ahead and focus on that earlier time and ask the same series of questions about that incident.

When all decisions made at that earliest time have been viewed, the person will feel relieved and more extroverted and it is then time to end the procedure.

If you feel the emotional reactions of your friend or loved one are extreme, use the list of resources in the appendix to find professional help. For the family that has strong ties to a religious group, there is often pastoral counseling available. For those who don't, many wonderful counseling centers exist where help can be obtained. The appendix of the book contains resources for obtaining such professional help.

Trauma of Humiliation

Helping a friend or loved one recover from a sense of humiliation can be tricky since it is often embarrassing or uncomfortable for the person to talk about the subject. It is well worth making the effort, however, as a humiliating incident can have a devastating effect on someone's life.

If you care for someone who is suffering this kind of humiliation, use the procedure that follows to help him or her begin a recovery.

Compassion Remedy

The first step in handling the emotional trauma of a feeling of humiliation is to let the person talk about when he or she first began to feel that way. Some encouragement may be needed at first. You can encourage a person to say more by use of the following prompts:

1. Tell me what happened.

2. Did anything else happen?

3. Is there anything else you want to tell me about that?

At no time during the conversation should you become critical or judgmental.

Example:

Marge had worked as a supervisor for 25 years and had always done a competent job. She had learned her skills on the job and her experience had been considered invaluable. When new management took over the corporation where she was employed, Marge was demoted to being an assistant to the new supervisor, a younger person with a brand new college degree in management. Marge was suffering the daily humiliation of watching someone with a fraction of her experience and skill take her place.

During that period of time, Marge's health began to suffer, her confidence plummeted, and her friends noticed that she had appeared to age at least ten years, a fact that was caused by the new lines of bitterness etched in her face. The blow to her confidence made it difficult for her to seek work elsewhere so she could end the intolerable work situation. When she finally was helped to express all that humiliation and bitterness by a compassionate friend, her confidence rose and she was able at last to find another more agreeable position.

Make a point of always letting the person know that you have heard what he or she is saying. A simple "uh huh" or "ok" is enough to acknowledge that you have heard someone. Most people will be very eager to talk to you as long as you remain compassionate and interested. You encourage the person to communicate fully by avoiding judgmental or critical communication or attitudes and by following the Golden Rules of Emotional First Aid. The person's recounting of the event may run for a few minutes or several hours. Be prepared to listen patiently throughout. If the person has told you about the incident but still has attention on it, ask him or her to tell you about it again one or more times.

Frequently, after telling you about the event, the person feels relieved and has no further interest in the event. If that is the case, end the Compassion Remedy at that point. If that is not the case, ask the person if there is something he or she now feels could be done about the event or if he or she now sees some way to handle the effects of the event in a positive manner. Looking at this point of view may help the person feel able to act as cause in the event rather than feeling victimized by it.

Check also for any decisions the person might have made at the time of the incident. Often someone makes major decisions during a time of stress and it is beneficial to take note of those decisions and to talk about them to a friend or loved one. Sometimes the decisions were wise ones and the talk reinforces them, but there are other times when the decisions would have proved to be destructive. An example might be a person who decides he or she is worthless because of the humiliation. If left unexamined, that decision could prove to be harmful. Once the person has had the chance to talk about the upset at length and to begin the healing process, he or she might change his or her mind about the wisdom of such a decision. The spotting of decisions and communication about them with a compassionate listener is one of the most beneficial parts of this procedure. There may be one decision or many. Take plenty of time on this question and give the person the chance to examine all decisions.

If, during the course of doing this procedure, the person starts to speak of an earlier similar upset, go ahead and focus on that earlier time and ask the same series of questions about that incident.

When all decisions made at that earliest time have been viewed, the person will feel relieved and more extroverted and it is then time to end the procedure.

If you feel the emotional reactions of your friend or loved one are extreme, use the list of resources in the appendix to find professional help. For the family that has strong ties to a religious group, there is often pastoral counseling available. For those who don't, many wonderful counseling centers exist where help can be obtained. The appendix of the book contains resources for obtaining such professional help.

Trauma of a Serious Physical Illness

A friend or loved one who is seriously physically ill needs medical help first and foremost, but there is often benefit to be gained from addressing the emotional trauma of such an illness too. Few doctors would disagree that a person's recovery will be speeded by the relief obtained from communicating to a compassionate listener about the fears, concerns, and considerations related to the illness.

If you have a friend or loved one who has experienced a serious physical illness, you may be able to offer him or her help by using the following procedures.

Once the immediate medical help has been given, the Calming Procedure may be helpful.

Calming Procedure

As noted in the introduction to this section, there are actions that can be taken in life to help those who are suffering a major illness. Do as many of these actions as it is possible for you to do.

❑ Help create a calm, quiet, predictable environment for the traumatized person

Example:

Bret had been ill with Cystic Fibrosis all of his life. Though advances had been made in treatment since he was first diagnosed, Bret had spent most of his life feeling that a death sentence was hanging over his head. He had watched other patients die and had feared for his own life on many occasions.

Although his life expectancy had improved because of medical advances and might continue to improve further, Bret had trouble focusing on his education for a future that he had long believed didn't exist. In addition, his doctors felt that the stress of his fears made him respond poorly to his medication. When Bret finally received help in dealing with his emotions and attitudes regarding his illness, his attitude toward his education became more focused and he took more pleasure in it. At that point, he also began to respond as the doctors had hoped to his medical treatment.

❑ Encourage the person to get extra nutritional support (stress burns more nutrients)

❏ Treat the person as gently as possible recognizing that an emotional injury is as destructive as a physical one

❏ Give as much physical contact as appropriate and acceptable: hugs, hand holding, pats on the shoulder, etc.

❏ Be reassuring whenever possible but don't attempt to make less of the loss or try to talk the person out of his or her feelings

❏ Help provide the presence of a compassionate adult until the worst of the trauma has passed

❏ Provide as much unconditional love as you can

When the preceding remedy is done, check with the person's physician to find out whether the ill person's stamina is great enough to allow for a session of several hours duration. It is sometimes necessary, when someone is ill, to break the procedure down into several days work. When your loved one's stamina is sufficient, begin the Compassion Remedy that follows, always watching carefully for signs of excessive fatigue and ending for the day if those signs appear.

Compassion Remedy

The first step in handling the emotional trauma of a serious illness is to let the person talk about when he or she first began to realize that he or she was ill and then continue with the full story. Some encouragement may be needed at first. You can encourage a person to say more by use of the following prompts:

1. Tell me what happened.

2. Did anything else happen?

3. Is there anything else you want to tell me about that?

At no time during the conversation should you become critical or judgmental. Make a point of always letting the person know that you have heard what he or she is saying. A simple "uh huh" or "ok" is enough to acknowledge that you have heard someone. Most people will be very eager to talk to you as long as you remain compassionate and interested. You encourage the person to communicate fully by avoiding judgmental or critical communication or attitudes and by following the Golden Rules of Emotional First Aid. The person's recounting of the event may run for a few minutes or several hours. Be prepared to listen patiently throughout. If the person has told you about the incident but still has attention on it, ask him or her to tell you about it again one or more times.

Frequently, after telling you about the event, the person feels relieved and has no further interest in the event. If that is the case, end the Compassion Remedy at that point. If that is not the case, ask the person if there is something he or she now feels could be done about the event or if he or she now sees some way to handle the effects of the event in a positive manner. Looking at this point of view may help the person feel able to act as cause in the event rather than feeling victimized by it.

Check also for any decisions the person might have made at the time of the illness. Often someone makes major decisions during a time of stress and it is beneficial to take note of those decisions and to talk about them to a friend or loved one. Sometimes the decisions were wise ones and the talk reinforces them, but there are other times when the decisions would have proved to be destructive. An example might be a person who decides he or she must always be very careful and avoid any activity that might lead to another illness. If left unexamined, that decision could prove to be harmful. Once the person has had the chance to talk about the upset at length and to begin the healing process, he or she might change his or her mind about the wisdom of such a decision. The spotting of decisions and communication about them with a compassionate listener is one of the most beneficial parts of this procedure. There may be one decision or many. Take plenty of time on this question and give the person the chance to examine all decisions.

If, during the course of doing this procedure, the person starts to speak of an earlier similar upset, go ahead and focus on that earlier time and ask the same series of questions about that incident.

When all decisions made at that earliest time have been viewed, the person will feel relieved and more extroverted and it is then time to end the procedure.

If you feel the emotional reactions of your friend or loved one are extreme, use the list of resources in the appendix to find professional help. For the family that has strong ties to a religious group, there is often pastoral counseling available. For those who don't, many wonderful counseling centers exist where help can be obtained. The appendix contains resources for obtaining such professional help.

Trauma of an Accident

A friend or loved one who has had a serious accident has often suffered emotional trauma as well. Fear is a common result of an accident as well as loss of trust, anxiety, anger, and a host of other emotions.

Right after the accident, as soon as medical help has been given, the Calming Procedure that follows can be done.

Calming Procedure

As noted in the introduction to this section, there are actions that can be taken in life to help those who are suffering the effects of an accident. Do as many of these actions as it is possible for you to do.

❏ Help create a calm, quiet, predictable environment for the traumatized person

❏ Encourage the person to get extra nutritional support (stress burns more nutrients)

❏ Treat the person as gently as possible recognizing that an emotional injury is as destructive as a physical one

Example:

Bill was an excellent skier who was also very careful and he'd never been injured on the slopes. One day, however, he skied over a patch of snow that appeared normal from the top. It covered a wide hole that gave way as he crossed over it. Bill's leg was broken in three places and his confidence in his ability to spot dangerous situations was shattered. Long after the leg had healed and he could have resumed skiing, Bill was too anxious to make the attempt. This anxiety, and his inability to overcome it, further reduced his confidence and damaged his self-esteem.

It wasn't until Bill sought emotional help that he was able to return to a sport he loved. The process of re-experiencing the incident repeatedly made him realize there was no error in his judgment or any lack of caution, merely a fluke that was very unlikely to be repeated. He also realized the he'd made a decision as he lay on his back waiting for medical help and in great pain. He had decided that he couldn't trust his power of observation well enough to continue skiing. With that decision uncovered, he was able to revise it and resume skiing.

❏ Give as much physical contact as appropriate and acceptable: hugs, hand holding, pats on the shoulder, etc.

❐ Be reassuring whenever possible, but don't attempt to make less of the loss or try to talk the person out of his or her feelings

❐ Help provide the presence of a compassionate adult until the worst of the trauma has passed

❐ Provide as much unconditional love as you can

When the preceding procedure is done, check with the person's physician to find out whether the person's stamina is great enough to allow for a session of several hours duration. It is sometimes necessary, when someone has had an accident, to break the procedure down into several days work. When your loved one's stamina is sufficient, begin the Compassion Remedy that follows, always watching carefully for signs of excessive fatigue and ending for the day if those signs appear.

Compassion Remedy

The first step in handling the emotional trauma of an accident is to let the person talk about when he or she first began to realize that an accident was about to occur and then continue to the end of the story. Some encouragement may be needed at first. You can encourage a person to say more by use of the following prompts:

1. Tell me what happened.

2. Did anything else happen?

3. Is there anything else you want to tell me about that?

At no time during the conversation should you become critical or judgmental. Make a point of always letting the person know that you have heard what he or she is saying. A simple "uh huh" or "ok" is enough to acknowledge that you have heard someone. Most people will be very eager to talk to you as long as you remain compassionate and interested. You encourage the person to communicate fully by avoiding judgmental or critical communication or attitudes and by following the Golden Rules of Emotional First Aid. The person's recounting of the event may run for a few minutes or several hours. Be prepared to listen patiently throughout. If the person has told you about the incident but still has attention on it, ask him or her to tell you about it again one or more times.

Frequently, after telling you about the event, the person feels relieved and has no further interest in the event. If that is the case, end the Compassion Remedy at that point. If that is not the case, ask the person if there is something he or she now feels could be done about the event or if he or she now sees some way to handle the effects of the event in a positive manner. Looking at this point of view may help the person feel able to act as cause in the event rather than feeling victimized by it.

Check also for any decisions the person might have made at the time of the accident. Often someone makes major decisions during a time of stress and it is beneficial to take note of those decisions and to talk about them to a friend or loved one. Sometimes the decisions were wise ones and the talk reinforces them, but there are other times when the decisions would have proved to be destructive. An example might be a person who decides he or she must become very cautious in order to never have it happen again. If left unexamined, that decision could prove to be harmful. Once the person has had the chance to talk about the upset at length and to begin the healing process, he or she might change his or her mind about the wisdom of such a decision. The spotting of decisions and communication about them with a compassionate listener is one of the most beneficial parts of this procedure. There may be one decision or many. Take plenty of time on this question and give the person the chance to examine all decisions.

If, during the course of doing this procedure, the person starts to speak of an earlier similar accident, go ahead and focus on that earlier time and ask the same series of questions about that incident.

When all decisions made at that earliest time have been viewed, the person will feel relieved and more extroverted and it is then time to end the procedure.

If you feel the emotional reactions of your friend or loved one are extreme, use the list of resources in the appendix to find professional help. For the family that has strong ties to a religious group, there is often pastoral counseling available. For those who don't, many wonderful counseling centers exist where help can be obtained. The appendix contains information on resources for obtaining such professional help.

Loss of a Body Part

There must be some sort of genetically imprinted concept of what the human body should look like because even tiny infants cry and show other signs of distress when shown a picture of a human body that has parts missing, scrambled, or distorted. It is no wonder, then, that we all react so strongly to losing a part of our body. Even the loss of a part that can be eliminated and still cause no threat to our survival—like a finger or toe—can cause tremendous emotional upset to the person who loses it. The loss of a body part that does impair our function, like a leg or an eye, can be an emotionally shattering incident.

> *Example:*
>
> *Sylvia lost the two outside fingers of her left hand in an industrial accident. Although she was still able to do her job well and to participate in all her former activities, and although the surgeon had done an outstanding job of reducing the scaring and leaving a smooth covering for the outside portion of her hand, Sylvia had a terrible time coming to grips with her loss. The reassurance of her family and friends that the sight of her hand was in no way repugnant did nothing to comfort her, and her confidence and self-esteem plummeted as depression took hold.*
>
> *It was a talk with her minister that finally opened the door to her healing. Sylvia recalled feeling repulsed by the sight of a child with only one hand when she was in the first grade. Her shock at that early age over the incomplete physical structure, and decisions she had made at that time about preferring death to being incomplete, were behind the inability to cope with her current loss. Compassionate communication about those fears helped her overcome them and get on with her life.*

If you have a friend or loved one who has suffered such a loss, use the Compassion Remedy that follows to help him or her begin to recover emotionally.

Compassion Remedy

The first step in handling the emotional trauma of losing a body part is to let the person talk about when he or she first began to realize that the loss would occur and then tell the whole story. Some encouragement may be needed at first. You can encourage a person to say more by use of the following prompts:

1. Tell me what happened.

2. Did anything else happen?

3. Is there anything else you want to tell me about that?

At no time during the conversation should you become critical or judgmental. Make a point of always letting the person know that you have heard what he or she is saying. A simple "uh huh" or "ok" is enough to acknowledge that you have heard someone. Most people will be very eager to talk to you as long as you remain compassionate and interested. You encourage the person to communicate fully by avoiding judgmental or critical communication or attitudes and by following the Golden Rules of Emotional First Aid. The person's recounting of the event may run for a few minutes or several hours. Be prepared to listen patiently throughout. If the person has told you about the incident but still has attention on it, ask him or her to tell you about it again one or more times.

Frequently, after telling you about the event, the person feels relieved and has no further interest in the event. If that is the case, end the Compassion Remedy at that point. If that is not the case, ask the person if there is something he or she now feels could be done about the event or if he or she now sees some way to handle the effects of the event in a positive manner. Looking at this point of view may help the person feel able to act as cause in the event rather than feeling victimized by it.

Check also for any decisions the person might have made at the time of the incident. Often someone makes major decisions during a time of stress and it is beneficial to take note of those decisions and to talk about them to a friend or loved one. Sometimes the decisions were wise ones and the talk reinforces them, but there are other times when the decisions would have proved to be destructive. An example might be a person who decides he or she is too deformed to ever be happy again. If left unexamined, that decision could prove to be harmful. Once the person has had the chance to talk about the upset at length and to begin the healing process, he or she might change his or her mind about the wisdom of such a decision. The spotting of decisions and communication about them with a compassionate listener is one of the most beneficial parts of this procedure. There may be one decision or many. Take plenty of time on this question and give the person the chance to examine all decisions.

If, during the course of doing this procedure, the person starts to speak of an earlier similar upset, go ahead and focus on that earlier time and ask the same series of questions about that incident.

When all decisions made at that earliest time have been viewed, the person will feel relieved and more extroverted and it is then time to end the procedure.

If you feel the emotional reactions of your friend or loved one are extreme, use the list of resources in the appendix to find professional help. For the family that has strong ties to a religious group, there is often pastoral counseling available. For those who don't, many wonderful counseling centers exist where help can be obtained. The appendix contains resources for obtaining such professional help.

Trauma of Physical or Sexual Abuse

Because the effects of physical and sexual abuse can be so devastating, our first recommendation is that you do everything in your power to help your friend or loved one get professional help. There are numerous support groups for this trauma and many of them are listed in the appendix. Most can recommend professionals who specialize in the treatment of physical and sexual abuse. The absolute first requirement, if the abuse is current, is to get your friend or loved one out of the dangerous environment and into a safe place. The groups listed in the appendix can also help you find out what your area of the world has to offer in terms of help in this action. More and more locations have shelters for abused/battered individuals.

On occasion, family or friends of abused individuals are frustrated by the fact that it seems impossible to get their loved ones to take the action required to get professional help, or there is some circumstance that prevents it. In those cases, you can do the remedies that follow to help your loved one. Often, after these remedies have been applied, the person will be more willing to seek professional help.

The procedures below can be done successfully by a friend

Example:

Wanda had grown up in a home where physical and sexual abuse were common. Her alcoholic father had regularly terrorized his family with his violence. As so often happens, Wanda, who had received no emotional help, married a man much like her father. When Kitty, Wanda's friend, saw her with bruises and burns, she tried to get Wanda to seek help.

A lifetime of emotional damage had made Wanda feel unworthy of such help. She refused to seek it, even going so far as to bail her husband out of jail when a neighbor had called the police after his latest attack. Kitty got a quick lesson in compassionate communication from her own therapist and bravely decided to try to provide the help herself. She was able to do well enough to raise Wanda's opinion of herself to the point where she finally sought shelter and professional help.

Though many years of continued help were necessary for Wanda's complete recovery, there is no doubt that it was Kitty's love and communication that started her on the path.

or family member who follows the instructions and the Golden Rules for Emotional First Aid carefully.

Calming Procedure

As noted in the introduction to this section, there are actions that can be taken in life to help someone who has suffered. Do as many of these actions as it is possible for you to do.

- ❏ Help create a calm, quiet, predictable environment for the traumatized person.

- ❏ Encourage the person to get extra nutritional support (stress burns more nutrients).

- ❏ Treat the person as gently as possible recognizing that an emotional injury is as destructive as a physical one.

- ❏ Give as much physical contact as appropriate and acceptable: hugs, hand holding, pats on the shoulder, etc.

- ❏ Be reassuring whenever possible but don't attempt to make less of the loss or try to talk the person out of his or her feelings.

- ❏ Help provide the presence of a compassionate adult until the worst of the trauma has passed.

- ❏ Provide as much unconditional love as you can

Once the procedure above has been done, continue with the Compassion Remedy that follows.

Compassion Remedy

The first step in helping with the emotional trauma of physical and sexual abuse is to let the person talk about when he or she first began to experience it and have them move forward telling the whole story. Some encouragement may be needed at first. You can encourage a person to say more by use of the following prompts:

1. Tell me what happened.

2. Did anything else happen?

3. Is there anything else you want to tell me about that?

At no time during the conversation should you become critical or judgmental. Make a point of always letting the person know that you have heard what he or she is saying. A simple "uh huh" or "ok" is enough to acknowledge that you have heard someone. Most people will be very eager to talk to you as long as you remain compassionate and interested. You encourage the person to communicate fully by avoiding judgmental or critical communication or attitudes and by following the Golden Rules of Emotional First Aid. The person's recounting of the event may run for a few minutes or several hours. Be prepared to listen patiently throughout. If the person has told you about the incident but still has attention on it, ask him or her to tell you about it again one or more times.

Frequently, after telling you about the event, the person feels relieved and has no further interest in the event. If that is the case, end the Compassion Remedy at that point. If that is not the case, ask the person if there is something he or she now feels could be done about the event or if he or she now sees some way to handle the effects of the event in a positive manner. Looking at this point of view may help the person feel able to act as cause in the event rather than feeling victimized by it.

Check also for any decisions the person might have made at the time of the incident. Often someone makes major decisions during a time of stress and it is beneficial to take note of those decisions and to talk about them to a friend or loved one. Sometimes the decisions were wise ones and the talk reinforces them, but there are other times when the decisions would have proved to be destructive. An example might be a person who decides he or she is worthless because of the abuse. If left unexamined, that decision could prove to be harmful. Once the person has had the chance to talk about the upset at length and to begin the healing process, he or she might change his or her mind about the wisdom of such a decision. The spotting of decisions and communication about them with a compassionate listener is one of the most beneficial parts of this procedure. There may be one decision or many. Take plenty of time on this question and give the person the chance to examine all decisions.

If, during the course of doing this procedure, the person starts to speak of an earlier similar upset, go ahead and focus on that earlier time and ask the same series of questions about that incident.

When all decisions made at that earliest time have been viewed, the person will feel relieved and more extroverted and it is then time to end the procedure.

Often, after this remedy is done, the person is more willing to seek further help from a professional who can guide his or her progress in a complete recovery.

If you feel the emotional reactions of your friend or loved one are extreme, use the list of resources in the appendix to find professional help. For the family that has strong ties to a religious group, there is often pastoral counseling available. For those who don't, many wonderful counseling centers exist where help can be obtained. The appendix contains resources for obtaining such professional help.

Loss caused by a Natural Disaster

The news seems always to be full of tales of floods, earthquakes, tornadoes, and other natural disasters. The focus of the stories is often on the death and the property damage, but the emotional trauma of the survivors is frequently devastating. Certainly events like Hurricane Katrina make that point. There is a Section in the book that addresses helping others in groups after a disaster (Section Five) but it can also be beneficial to help individuals who are victims of catastrophic events. Additionally, the local mental health resources can be tremendously overburdened in the case of a widespread disaster.

There is a great deal we can do to help each other while the professionals deal with the most serious or difficult cases. Some of the indicators that a friend or loved one has suffered emotional trauma include the following:

❒ Depression that can begin almost immediately after the disaster but that often does not show up until weeks or months later

❒ A fixation on the disaster that is apparent in conversation

❒ Feelings of guilt for having survived when others didn't or for having more minor losses when others experienced major ones

❒ Anxiety and an inability to get on with life

❒ Bad dreams and flashbacks of the disaster

❒ Fears and phobias associated with the disaster

The Compassion Remedy that follows is one way to give effective help to a friend or loved one who is suffering the effects of trauma due to a natural disaster.

Compassion Remedy

The first step in handling the emotional trauma of a natural disaster is to let the person talk about when he or she first realized the disaster had struck and then follow through with the whole story beginning to end. Some encouragement may be needed at first.

You can encourage a person to say more by use of the following prompts:

1. Tell me what happened.

2. Did anything else happen?

3. Is there anything else you want to tell me about that?

At no time during the conversation should you become critical or judgmental. Make a point of always letting the person know that you have heard what he or she is saying. A simple "uh huh" or "ok" is enough to acknowledge that you have heard someone. Most people will be very eager to talk to you as long as you remain compassionate and interested. You encourage the person to communicate fully by avoiding judgmental or critical communication or attitudes and by following the Golden Rules of Emotional First Aid. The person's recounting of the event may run for a few minutes or several hours. Be prepared to listen patiently throughout. If the person has told you about the incident but still has attention on it, ask him or her to tell you about it again one or more times.

Frequently, after telling you about the event, the person feels relieved and has no further interest in the event. If that is the case, end the Compassion Remedy at that point. If that is not the case, ask the person if there is something he or she now feels could be done about the event or if he or she now sees some way to handle the effects of the event in a positive manner. Looking at this point of view may help the person feel able to act as cause in the event rather than feeling victimized by it.

Check also for any decisions the person might have made at the time of the incident. Often someone makes major decisions during a time of stress and it is beneficial to take note of those decisions and to talk about them to a friend or loved one. Sometimes the decisions were wise ones and the talk reinforces them, but there are other times when the decisions would have proved to be destructive. An example might be a person who decides he or she has nowhere to hide from such a disaster and so must be constantly on guard. If left unexamined, that decision could prove to be harmful. Once the person has had the chance to talk about the upset at length and to begin the healing process, he or she might change his or her mind about the wisdom of such a decision. The spotting of decisions and communication about them with a compassionate listener is one of the most beneficial parts of this procedure. There may be one decision or many. Take plenty of time on this question and give the person the chance to examine all decisions.

If, during the course of doing this procedure, the person starts to speak of an earlier similar upset, go ahead and focus on that earlier time and ask the same series of questions about that incident.

When all decisions made at that earliest time have been viewed, the person will feel relieved and more extroverted and it is then time to end the procedure.

If you feel the emotional reactions of your friend or loved one are extreme, use the list of resources in the appendix to find professional help. For the family that has strong ties to a religious group, there is often pastoral counseling available. For those who don't, many wonderful counseling centers exist where help can be obtained. The appendix contains resources for obtaining such professional help.

Loss of Youth or Physical Attractiveness

Why can some people accept the loss of their youth or their physical attractiveness without any real feeling of upset while others find it to be a traumatizing experience? Most mental health professionals feel it has to do with what we base our self-esteem upon. A person who, due to decisions made early in his or her upbringing, feels that his or her value in life is based upon an attractive and youthful appearance will find the loss of that youth or attractive appearance a frightening and threatening event. Another individual who bases his or her self-esteem on wisdom gained or accumulated experience will not be as bothered by the end of youthfulness.

Obviously it would be best if we all based our self-esteem on things that are not transitory, like our uniqueness as human beings, for we would never suffer the loss of that esteem if we were able to do so. A large part of the help you give your friend or loved one in the procedure that follows will result from the encouragement you offer him or her to re-examine those early decisions.

The loss of youth or physical attractiveness are not always tied together. Is the loss of physical attractiveness serious enough to be listed in a volume dedicated to helping people deal with trauma? Most of us would not categorize that loss as a trauma, especially if it is the gradual diminishment that sometimes occurs with

Example:

Sarah received only one form of praise and approval as a child. Her parents overlooked completely her loving nature, her sharp mind, and her sense of humor, and focused instead on her appearance. She was complimented frequently for the beauty of her skin, the richness of her thick wavy hair, and her slender youthful figure. It was not surprising that Sarah felt a panic as she approached middle age and her skin lost its youthful sheen, her hair thinned a bit and turned gray, and her figure became harder to maintain.

Sarah's decision as a child that she had only one area of value prevented her from noticing the beneficial effects of her education, experience, and maturity. She saw the passage of time as a threat to any feeling of value or pleasure and became increasingly depressed as the years went by. When she spotted this destructive decision during the Compassion Remedy, she was then able to confront the process of aging with a more positive attitude.

age. A sudden loss, however, or even a gradual loss to a person who bases his or her self-esteem upon that physical attractiveness, can be traumatic and it deserves to be dealt with seriously.

If you have a friend or loved one who shows concern over a loss of physical attractiveness, don't make the mistake of taking it lightly and trying to handle it with just a reassurance that he or she looks fine. Instead apply the Compassion Remedy that follows and help that person get to the bottom of the problem.

If we become impatient with our loved ones about the "shallowness" of taking the loss of youth hard, or if we go into agreement with the idea that there is something tragic about it, then we will lose our ability to help. Instead, we need to feel compassion for someone who bases his or her self-esteem on such a transitory quality and encourage that person to communicate his or her feelings of loss fully so that there will be relief from the pain. It is also wise to encourage that friend or loved one to seek further help in learning to find new ways to increase self-esteem.

Compassion Remedy

The first step in handling the emotional trauma of loss of youth is to ask about when the person first began to feel that he or she was becoming less valuable due to the loss of his or her youth. Some encouragement may be needed at first. You can encourage a person to say more by use of the following prompts:

1. Tell me what happened.
2. Did anything else happen?
3. Is there anything else you want to tell me about that?

At no time during the conversation should you become critical or judgmental. Make a point of always letting the person know that you have heard what he or she is saying. A simple "uh huh" or "ok" is enough to acknowledge that you have heard someone. Most people will be very eager to talk to you as long as you remain compassionate and interested. You encourage the person to communicate fully by avoiding judgmental or critical communication or attitudes and by following the Golden Rules of Emotional First Aid.

The person's recounting of the event may run for a few minutes or several hours. Be prepared to listen patiently throughout. If the person has told you about the incident but still has attention on it, ask him or her to tell you about it again one or more times.

Frequently, after telling you about the event, the person feels relieved and has no further interest in the event. If that is the case, end the Compassion Remedy at that point. If that is not the case, ask the person if there is something he or she now feels could be done about the event or if he or she now sees some way to handle the effects of the event in a positive manner. Looking at this point of view may help the person feel able to act as cause in the event rather than feeling victimized by it.

Check also for any decisions the person might have made at the time of the incident. Often someone makes major decisions during a time of stress and it is beneficial to take note of those decisions and to talk about them to a friend or loved one. Sometimes the decisions were wise ones and the talk reinforces them, but there are other times when the decisions would have proved to be destructive. An example might be a person who decides he or she is worthless because of the loss. If left unexamined, that decision could prove to be harmful. Once the person has had the chance to talk about the upset at length and to begin the healing process, he or she might change his or her mind about the wisdom of such a decision. The spotting of decisions and communication about them with a compassionate listener is one of the most beneficial parts of this procedure. There may be one decision or many. Take plenty of time on this question and give the person the chance to examine all decisions.

If, during the course of doing this procedure, the person starts to speak of an earlier similar upset, go ahead and focus on that earlier time and ask the same series of questions about that incident.

When all decisions made at that earliest time have been viewed, the person will feel relieved and more extroverted and it is then time to end the procedure.

If you feel the emotional reactions of your friend or loved one are extreme, use the list of resources in the appendix to find professional help. For the family that has strong ties to a religious group, there is often pastoral counseling available. For those who don't, many wonderful counseling centers exist where help can be obtained. The appendix contains resources for obtaining such professional help.

Trauma of an Unintentional Harmful Act

The trauma caused by the commission of an unintentional harmful act is sometimes underestimated. The fact that we're upset by our unintentional, harmful acts has its roots deep in the foundation of our life. Underlying it is the cornerstone of mankind's basic goodness. This goodness is very hard to see in some people and it's no wonder that many of us begin to doubt its existence. Anyone who has worked with people to help them confront the most traumatic parts of their life, however, is aware of the fact that as they unburden themselves of the pain, their activities become directed more and more toward survival rather than destruction. You don't have to beat people into being better people or talk them into it. It's a natural evolution that occurs as they resolve the traumatic incidents in their life.

Because people are basically good, they are very affected by

> *Example:*
>
> *Three-year-old Tommy is left alone one day in the kitchen while he's having lunch. He realizes that by pouring his pudding out on the floor, he can make wonderful patterns and designs, something which he considers aesthetically pleasing. Because he's very young, he has no idea that it's hard to get chocolate pudding out of the carpet in the dining area. He's having a wonderful time creating this masterpiece.*
>
> *Then mom comes into the room and screams in horror as she views her rug. She seems harmed by what has been done as she expresses upset at the work that will be involved in cleaning the spots out of the rug. Tommy sees this person, whom he loves more than anyone and depends upon for his survival, in tears over the damage that has been done. He is horrified. He never intended to hurt his mother. He has just committed an unintentional harmful act. This incident, which his mother had long since forgotten, led to a decision by Tommy that the world was an unpredictable and dangerous place.*

the unintentional harmful acts they've committed. It's never the desire of a small child to harm someone. In fact, committing an unintentional harmful act is one of life's most upsetting experiences. It often takes far longer to handle the effects of the unintentional harmful act done to someone else than it would to handle the effect of a harmful act done by another to oneself.

Because we're basically good—when we've hurt someone and we don't understand why or can't be certain we'll be able to avoid repeating the act—one way to guarantee we can avoid that situation in the future is to limit our power. Because of this, the result of this type of traumatic incident is often that the person becomes fearful and anxious about life and is very introverted or withdrawn.

These unintentional harmful acts can range from minor acts, like the child who decorates the dining room with pudding, to a very serious act like forgetting to lock the gate to the swimming pool and having a child enter it and drown. Even when the results have been disastrous, the person deserves to receive our help. Most of us have made mistakes that could have led to disaster but we were fortunate and the potential for disaster did not turn to reality.

Compassion Remedy

The first step in handling the emotional trauma of having committed a harmful act is to let the person talk about when he or she first began to feel that he or she had caused great harm and then continue with the whole story. Some encouragement may be needed at first. You can encourage a person to say more by use of the following prompts:

1. Tell me what happened.

2. Did anything else happen?

3. Is there anything else you want to tell me about that?

At no time during the conversation should you become critical or judgmental. Make a point of always letting the person know that you have heard what he or she is saying. A simple "uh huh" or "ok" is enough to acknowledge that you have heard someone. Most people will be very eager to talk to you as long as you remain compassionate and interested. You encourage the person to communicate fully by avoiding judgmental or critical communication or attitudes and by following the Golden Rules of Emotional First Aid. The person's recounting of the event may run for a few minutes or several hours. Be prepared to listen patiently throughout. If the person has told you about the incident but still has attention on it, ask him or her to tell you about it again one or more times.

Frequently, after telling you about the event, the person feels relieved and has no further interest in the event. If that is the case, end the Compassion Remedy at that point. If that is not the case, ask the person if there is something he or she now feels could be done about the event or if he or she now sees some way to handle the effects of the event in a positive manner. Looking at this point of view may help the person feel able to act as cause in the event rather than feeling victimized by it.

Check also for any decisions the person might have made at the time of the incident. Often someone makes major decisions during a time of stress and it is beneficial to take note of those decisions and to talk about them to a friend or loved one. Sometimes the decisions were wise ones and the talk reinforces them, but there are other times when the decisions would have proved to be destructive. An example might be a person who decides to be very cautious in the future because he or she is unable to predict whey he or she might cause great harm. If left unexamined, that decision could prove to be harmful. Once the person has had the chance to talk about the upset at length and to begin the healing process, he or she might change his or her mind about the wisdom of such a decision. The spotting of decisions and communication about them with a compassionate listener is one of the most beneficial parts of this procedure. There may be one decision or many. Take plenty of time on this question and give the person the chance to examine all decisions.

If, during the course of doing this procedure, the person starts to speak of an earlier similar upset, go ahead and focus on that earlier time and ask the same series of questions about that incident.

When all decisions made at that earliest time have been viewed, the person will feel relieved and more extroverted and it is then time to end the procedure.

If you feel the emotional reactions of your friend or loved one are extreme, use the list of resources in the appendix to find profes-

Crisis of Faith

A crisis of faith for a devout person is a very real trauma. The term crisis of faith does not apply only to religion. A person can have a crisis of faith in mankind or in the goodness of others, for instance, or a crisis of faith in his or her family. Any person, group, ideal, or trait in which the person has had a feeling of faith (a job, an organization, a religion, an ability, a political system, etc.) can cause a crisis of faith if that bond of trust is broken.

Never underestimate the damage done when the faith of a friend or loved one is shattered. The procedure that follows is designed to help your loved one begin to regain his or her sense of well being after such a major disappointment.

Compassion Remedy

The first step in handling a crisis of faith is to let the person talk about when he or she first began to feel that his or her faith in someone or something was not justified. Some encouragement may be needed at first. You can encourage a person to say more by use of the following prompts:

Example:

Jenny had always placed great faith in the Senator for whom she had worked for the last 15 years. She felt he was a good, decent man who genuinely wanted the best for his constituents. Jenny went far and above the usual demands of the job, investing a great deal of her personal time and often sacrificing her private life for the needs of her boss.

When the Senator was proven to have accepted a bribe for his vote on an important issue, Jenny felt more than just betrayed. She felt a sense of hopeless about the nature of man that rendered her ill and broken in spirit.

Help given by a friend enabled her to spot the point where she had placed all her faith in a flawed human being and she was able to recover from the feeling of loss and lead a more balanced life.

1. Tell me what happened.

2. Did anything else happen?

3. Is there anything else you want to tell me about that?

At no time during the conversation should you become critical or judgmental. Make a point of always letting the person know that you have heard what he or she is saying. A simple "uh huh" or "ok" is enough to acknowledge that you have heard someone. Most people will be very eager to talk to you as long as you remain compassionate and interested. You encourage the person to communicate fully by avoiding judgmental or critical communication or attitudes and by following the Golden Rules of Emotional First Aid. The person's recounting of the event may run for a few minutes or several hours. Be prepared to listen patiently throughout. If the person has told you about the incident but still has attention on it, ask him or her to tell you about it again one or more times.

Frequently, after telling you about the event, the person feels relieved and has no further interest in the event. If that is the case, end the Compassion Remedy at that point. If that is not the case, ask the person if there is something he or she now feels could be done about the event or if he or she now sees some way to handle the effects of the event in a positive manner. Looking at this point of view may help the person feel able to act as cause in the event rather than feeling victimized by it.

> **Example:**
>
> *Tom had always felt that family could be counted upon, even when all else failed. He had great faith that, if he gave his all to the family, his family would be there for him if he was ever in need.*
>
> *When Tom had a serious stroke at the age of 55 and his wife and children, unable to deal with the physical demands of his nursing care, had him put in a care facility, he was crushed. His faith in the strength of the family unit came crashing down around him. The severe depression caused by this "crisis of faith" made his recovery far more difficult than expected.*
>
> *When he was able to spot the source of his basic beliefs, he was better able to accept the "human nature" of his family members.*

Check also for any decisions the person might have made at the time of the incident. Often someone makes major decisions during a time of stress and it is beneficial to take note of those decisions and to talk about them to a friend or loved one. Sometimes the decisions were wise ones and the talk reinforces them, but there are other times when the decisions would have proved to be destructive. An example might be a person who decides he or she can never have faith in anything again. If left unexamined, that decision could prove to be harmful. Once the person has had the chance to talk about the upset at length and to begin the healing process, he or she might change his or her mind about the wisdom of such a decision. The spotting of decisions and communication about them with a compassionate listener is one of the most beneficial parts of this procedure. There may be one decision or many. Take plenty of time on this question and give the person the chance to examine all decisions.

If, during the course of doing this procedure, the person starts to speak of an earlier similar upset, go ahead and focus on that earlier time and ask the same series of questions about that incident.

When all decisions made at that earliest time have been viewed, the person will feel relieved and more extroverted and it is then time to end the procedure.

If you feel the emotional reactions of your friend or loved one are extreme, use the appendix to find professional help. For the family that has strong ties to a religious group, there is often pastoral counseling available. For those who don't, many wonderful counseling centers exist where help can be obtained. The appendix of the book contains information on resources for obtaining such professional help.

Trauma due to Crime or Violence

Trauma resulting from crimes or violence goes well beyond the injuries inflicted or the property lost. There is an invasion of privacy factor as well as a violation of the personal sanctity of the person. This invasion and violation are often described by the victim as the most painful part of the incident. A loss of faith in the goodness of mankind is also frequently mentioned.

An act of crime or violence, even if injuries were minor or nonexistent and/or the material loss was insubstantial, should still be addressed. It is difficult for people who have endured such a crime to recover the peace of mind and happiness they enjoyed prior to the act. Likewise, someone who lives in what amounts to a war zone may also need help even if they haven't been attacked directly.

If you have a friend or loved one who shows any lingering effects from a crime or act of violence, use the Compassion Remedy that follows to help him or her recover.

Compassion Remedy

The first step in handling the emotional trauma resulting from crime or violence is to let the person talk about when he or she first began to realize there was a dangerous environment and then

> **Example:**
>
> Tom attended an inner-city school. He was under constant peer pressure to join in the gang activities that many of his friends had turned to lately. Only his strong family support had kept him from doing so. Violence had become so common that Tom planned his whole day—the routes he took to and from school, the locations where he ate lunch, etc.—so that he could avoid the threats. So many of his friends had been injured or killed that he had lost count.
>
> Tom had many of the symptoms of Post Traumatic Stress Disorder. His dreams were filled with the scenes of violence he'd witnessed. Certain locations where the violence had taken place caused flashbacks. He found it tremendously hard to focus on his studies. In many ways, he might as well have been the victim of a war, for his life and his neighborhood resembled a war zone.
>
> The Compassion Remedy can also be used in a situation like this where the violence happened to others and is a constant threat for someone like Tom.

continue by telling the whole story. Some encouragement may be needed at first. You can encourage a person to say more by use of the following prompts:

1. Tell me what happened.

2. Did anything else happen?

3. Is there anything else you want to tell me about that?

At no time during the conversation should you become critical or judgmental. Make a point of always letting the person know that you have heard what he or she is saying. A simple "uh huh" or "ok" is enough to acknowledge that you have heard someone. Most people will be very eager to talk to you as long as you remain compassionate and interested. You encourage the person to communicate fully by avoiding judgmental or critical communication or attitudes and by following the Golden Rules of Emotional First Aid. The person's recounting of the event may run for a few minutes or several hours. Be prepared to listen patiently throughout. If the person has told you about the incident but still has attention on it, ask him or her to tell you about it again one or more times.

> *Example:*
>
> *Cynthia was mugged one day as she walked home from the park with her children. She was knocked to the pavement, an act that caused minor injuries, and her purse was stolen.*
>
> *Long after the physical damage had healed, Cynthia was still too frightened to take her children outside. The world seemed a dark and sinister place. She mourned the loss of photos and sentimental items that had been in her purse far more than the small amounts of money that had been taken. She had difficulty trusting anyone, even her husband. It took an opportunity to communicate at great length with a compassionate friend before she began to trust again.*

Frequently, after telling you about the event, the person feels relieved and has no further interest in the event. If that is the case, end the Compassion Remedy at that point. If that is not the case, ask the person if there is something he or she now feels could be done about the event or if he or she now sees some way to handle the effects of the event in a positive manner. Looking at this point of view may help the person feel able to act as cause in the event rather than feeling victimized by it.

Check also for any decisions the person might have made at the time of the incident. Often someone makes major decisions during a time of stress and it is beneficial to take note of those decisions and to talk about them to a friend or loved one. Sometimes the decisions were wise ones and the talk reinforces them, but there are other times when the decisions would have proved to be destructive. An example might be a person who decides to hide out from the world because of the violence. If left unexamined, that decision could prove to be harmful. Once the person has had the chance to talk about the upset at length and to begin the healing process, he or she might change his or her mind about the wisdom of such a decision. The spotting of decisions and communication about them with a compassionate listener is one of the most beneficial parts of this procedure. There may be one decision or many. Take plenty of time on this question and give the person the chance to examine all decisions.

If, during the course of doing this procedure, the person starts to speak of an earlier similar upset, go ahead and focus on that earlier time and ask the same series of questions about that incident.

When all decisions made at that earliest time have been viewed, the person will feel relieved and more extroverted and it is then time to end the procedure.

If you feel the emotional reactions of your friend or loved one are extreme, use the list of resources in the appendix to find professional help. For the family that has strong ties to a religious group, there is often pastoral counseling available. For those who don't, many wonderful counseling centers exist where help can be obtained. The appendix of the book contains resources for obtaining such professional help.

Section Two—Childhood Traumas

Are there differences in how you might use the emotional first aid procedures with a child as opposed to an adult? Yes, of course there are! But they are minor ones. The **Seven Golden Rules of Emotional First Aid**, as noted in the chapter called **Vital Information**, are equally important when working with a child.

There are three primary differences between doing the procedures given in this book with a child rather than with an adult: one is the need to keep the role of parent or guardian completely separate from the role of listener; the second is the attention span of the child; and the third is the child's ability to communicate verbally.

1. Parent Versus Listener

Children must be treated with respect and be allowed to maintain their dignity. When you are helping a child through a traumatic incident, it's quite easy to lapse into the "normal" method of communication with children including lots of unsolicited advice. Don't ever succumb to the temptation to do this. The procedures that follow are not effective in the face of a violation of the **Seven Golden Rules**. Offer advice to a child at another time if you must, but don't do it while using the procedures in this section.

You will be able to help a child recover from the losses and traumas of life to the exact extent that you can offer him or her a compassionate, non-judgmental listener.

2. Attention Span

The age of the child will largely determine his or her attention span and your work with the child will need to accommodate this. However, children who are traumatized will sometimes be quite fixated on the incident causing the trauma and will frequently be able to focus much longer than normal when communicating about a traumatic incident. In fact, they may be able to focus on little else until they have been able to voice their fears.

As you do the procedures in this book, allow enough time to take the child to a point of completion. The child's interest is your best indicator of how long to address the issue. Never force a child to continue past the point when he or she has lost interest. Often the best indication you have that you have been able to help the child is the fact that his or her attention is no longer fixated on the incident and has returned to the present.

When you see that point reached, accept it as progress and let the child go out to play. Return to the subject only if you see new signs of fear or upset surfacing in the child.

3. Verbal Abilities of the Child

The procedures in this book are worded in a manner that is appropriate for a child eight or more years of age. Simplify the wording for a slightly younger child. A child must be able to communicate verbally to use the procedures. Four or five years of age is the earliest point when the Compassion Remedy would be effective with the exact age of effectiveness depending on the individual child's level of verbal skills. The Calming Procedure is effective for a child of any age.

Phases of a Trauma

There are four distinct phases a child goes through when he or she experiences a trauma. How much time is spent in each phase is determined largely by the quality of the help received by that child. The four stages are as follows:

1. Shock

The trauma victim may feel dazed or immobilized at times, have difficulty with his or her memory, or feel as though his or her sense of time is distorted. He or she is likely to feel angry, anxious, and frustrated. Physical reactions like nausea, muscle aches, and a pounding heart are common.

2. Denial

The trauma victim may begin to doubt what he or she saw and that it had any effect upon him or her. The child may feel emotionally numb and wish to isolate himself or herself from family and friends, or conversely be euphoric or "wired" and want to talk.

3. Impact

The full impact of the incident begins to sink in after the initial shock and denial have subsided. Often children have nightmares following a trauma and most have a difficult time sleeping for at least a few days. The child might feel preoccupied with thoughts about it during the day. In very strong trauma, brief lapses can occur when the child feels as if the incident is actually reoccurring. These "mini-flashbacks" can be particularly disturbing, and can make the victim feel as if he or she is "going crazy." He or she is not. These are all normal responses to abnormal events and should improve over time. The child may question how well he or she behaved during the disaster. The child may condemn himself or herself—or others—for not doing enough or obsess about "what if...." These self-doubts are common and expected. They are also very often exaggerated or unfounded. It's important for the child not to give in to such feelings of self-blame, rage, or depression by isolating himself or herself. This will only make things worse.

4. Resolution

Recovery from psychological traumatization is a painful, but natural process for most children. It is normal for a child who has been psychologically traumatized to need to talk about what happened — to parents, friends, clergy, counselors, etc. Especially valuable are talks with other children who have been through the same thing or something similar. They can understand what the trauma victim is experiencing. This is the reason support groups can be so helpful. The more the child talks about it with people who understand, the sooner the difficulties will pass.

When the child has some understanding of what the phases entail, it can be easier for him or her to deal with the trauma. It is important for that child to know that he or she is not alone in his or her feelings and is not going crazy but is having perfectly normal reactions. One of the techniques you will learn in this book is called an Orientation Remedy. It is designed to be done right at the scene of the trauma if necessary and it includes the information above as an educational step. The material will need to be simplified and explained, of course, at the level of understanding of the child.

For a child too young to verbalize, the best remedy for a traumatic incident is the Calming Procedure below.

Calming Procedure for a Child

Provide the child with as many of the following things as possible:

- A calm, quiet, predictable environment
- Extra nutritional support if needed (stress burns more nutrients)
- Very gentle handling
- Lots of physical contact: hugs, caresses, etc., as appropriate
- Lots of softly spoken reassurances (even a child who doesn't understand all the words will feel the intention behind them)
- Constant presence of a compassionate adult until the worst of the trauma has passed
- For a toddler, the chance to play act strong emotions using dolls
- The chance to vocalize rage or fear through crying, shouting, etc., without being told to be quiet
- Plenty of love!!!

Older children can also benefit from all the actions above in addition to the Compassion Remedy which follows at the end of this Section. The subject matter for a child's traumas can be slightly different than those for an adult. Following is a list of topics that describe the type of events a child would consider traumatic that an adult might not think of in quite the same way.

Loss of Confidence

Loss of a Classmate or Teacher

Violence in the School

Feelings of Failure

Humiliation

Abandonment

Feeling Stupid

Feeling Left Out

Betrayal

Serious Physical Illness

Medical Operation

Serious Accident

Loss of a Body Part Due to Physical Accident, Injury, or Illness

Physical/Sexual Abuse

Loss of a Parent, Grandparent, or Other Close Family Member

Loss of Stability Due to Divorce, Separation or Abandonment

Loss of a Home

Feeling Like a Disappointment

Feeling of Inferiority

False Accusations

Feeling Different

Loss of Security Due to Illness in the Family

Jealousy of a Sibling/New Baby

Here is some information on each of these areas that commonly are of concern to children.

Loss of Confidence

The loss of confidence in a child is always preceded by a traumatic event, one which the child considers overwhelming and which shook the child's faith in his or her ability to deal with the world. Always keep in mind that an event that an adult might consider minor can appear overwhelming to a child. How can you tell when your child's confidence has been damaged? Here are some warning signs.

❑ Sudden desire to stay home from school or after-school events

❑ Avoidance of friends and classmates that child had formerly welcomed

❑ Sudden increase in the amount of time spent sleeping or resting

❑ Giving up of formerly enjoyed hobbies, sports, or practices

❑ Sudden boastfulness (a sign of lack of confidence, not an excess of it)

❑ Moodiness in a formerly cheerful child

❑ Sudden need for frequent reassurance

❑ Clinging behavior in a formerly independent child

Example

Susan's mother noticed her daughter, a good student who always enjoyed school, suddenly didn't want to attend, cried easily, and seemed upset about doing her homework. Susan's mother commented on her observations in a manner that showed compassion and no hint of criticism.

"I've noticed you're not enjoying school as much these days, Honey. Did something happen to spoil the fun for you?"

"My handwriting is awful," Susan responded.

"What made you feel it was awful? Did someone say it was?" asked Susan's mom.

This question prompted a flood of tears and the statement, "They all laughed at me" from Susan.

For Susan the traumatic incident that needed to be addressed was the humiliation of being laughed at by the other children. Susan's mother may have considered that a minor event but she wisely treated it with great respect and ran the Compassion Remedy with Susan. The result was a renewal of Susan's enthusiasm for school.

A child with a chronic lack of self confidence may have traumatic incidents very early in life and will need professional assistance in regaining that confidence. A child with a reasonably high level of confidence who suddenly loses it may have a traumatic incident just preceding that drop and can usually be helped by a caring family member or friend.

The first step, of course, is in talking to the child and finding out what that traumatic incident was. A simple observation to the child is often enough to start the communication process. Then use the Children's Compassion Remedy at the end of this Section to help the child recover from the event.

Loss of a Classmate or Teacher

There are usually two reasons for the loss of a classmate or teacher. One is a move to a new school, or the move of his or her friend or teacher. The other is the loss through death or serious illness of a friend or teacher. The latter, of course, is likely to be the more traumatic of the two events, though neither situation should be taken lightly when it is causing distress to the child

The Compassion Remedy will help in either case. A note of warning, however. The child who takes the move to another school of a classmate extremely hard may need additional help. Such a close attachment to another student could indicate a shortage of friends or close relationships in general. In

Example

Six-year-old Tiffany took it very hard when her best friend, Emily, moved away with her family. Tiffany began to resist going to school each morning. Her mother took the time to have Tiffany communicate all about her sense of loss when Emily left. In the course of doing the Compassion Remedy, Tiffany's mother realized how important this one friend was to Tiffany because she was very shy.

Tiffany recovered from the loss with a combination of two actions that were taken. One was the chance to communicate fully to her mother. The other was the increased social activity her mother provided by allowing Tiffany to take dance lessons and attend group swimming activities.

Helping your children by using the Children's Compassion Remedy has the added benefit of making a parent fully aware of a child's feelings

such a case, parents may want to have a professional see the child to assess whether there are more serious underlying problems.

In most cases through, it is normal to feel upset at the loss of a favorite classmate, and the Children's Compassion Remedy at the end of this Section will help in the healing process.

Childhood Violence in the School

For some children, violence in the school is unfortunately a regular occurrence and the Children's Compassion Remedy at the end of this chapter may need to be done repeatedly. The only long-term solution for such a problem is to remove the child from such an environment and/or to enlist the aid of the other parents/teachers/officials in improving the school's security. An ideal society would have no violence in the schools but until we can achieve that ideal, it is unfortunately necessary to try to counteract the violence as much as possible.

A single or rare violent event is all too common these days and it's important for parents to realize that even when their child is not directly involved, such an event can have a lasting effect if it is not properly addressed. A child who feels the environment could be threatening will have more difficulty applying himself or herself to study.

A child of any age who has been exposed to violence needs lots of extra reassurance. Such a child can benefit from some of the actions mentioned in the Introduction to this section as part of the Calming Procedure. See the end of the Section for the exact steps of the procedure.

Even a violent event that was not directly witnessed by the child but is the subject of

> **Example**
>
> *When a 10-year-old boy was beaten by older boys on his way home from school, not only was the boy traumatized but so were his classmates who had observed or been told of the beating.*
>
> *More and more often today, schools are providing group trauma aid using techniques like the ones described in Section Five of this manual.*
>
> *It is still wise to work with the children on an individual basis too.*

conversation at school can be addressed. In such a case, it is the moment of hearing the stories of the violence that needs to be the topic for the Compassion Remedy at the end of this section.

Childhood Feelings of Failure

There is no sadder sight in life than a child who considers himself or herself a failure. Don't ever observe such a feeling in a child without acting to help. It is the accumulation of all of those moments of failure that rob a child of joy and send him or her on a downward path. If you even suspect that a child may be feeling such a loss, act quickly to remedy the situation.

Some of the common signs of a child who is feeling like a failure include the following:

- Lack of ability to look people in the eye
- A feeling of sadness
- An unwillingness to try new activities
- A listless, apathetic attitude
- A loss of self esteem

Prevention is the best path here and parents would be wise to monitor all activities carefully so that the gradient of difficulty is just right and the child can have a series of successes. This is not always within the parent's control however, and the feeling of failure can come from an activ-

> **Example**
>
> *Carol's father, Fred, used a phrase he had often heard from his parents as a child when his children had not done as he wished. He said, "I'm so disappointed in you."*
>
> *His two older children did not let this negative comment affect them a lot as they were by nature very confident, outgoing children. But Carol, a sensitive, quiet child who tried very hard to please, found her father's disappointment hard to confront. She became more and more quiet and sad as she failed again and again to win his approval.*
>
> *Fortunately, the family's minister was able to use the Children's Compassion Remedy to help Carol and he was also able to explain to her father what a devastating effect his comments were having on her. When Fred learned to discontinue use of a comment that he realized had also hurt him when he was a child, the whole family was happier.*

ity at school over which parents have little control. When the child seems to experience this feeling of failure frequently, it is time for a discussion with school personnel to learn what can be done to prevent it. There is never an excuse for allowing an activity to make a child feel a sense of failure. Even the most difficult action, learned at the proper gradient, can be a series of small wins.

To help a child who has begun to feel like a failure, use the Children's Compassion Remedy at the end of this Section of the manual.

Trauma of Humiliation

There are many different actions that can cause a child to feel a sense of humiliation. It is important for parents or guardians not to apply their own standards to the idea of what might cause a child to feel humiliated. The key is the child's own feelings.

A simple mishap like a momentary loss of bladder control in a young child may seem like a minor event to a parent, but it may represent a major trauma in the life of a child. Likewise, a sense of what is humiliating can vary from one child to another. The child who shrugs off the bladder control accident may instead feel traumatized by having to wear shabby clothing or by a loss at a game of volleyball.

A parent can determine when a child may be suffering the trauma of humiliation by the following signs:

- Sudden desire to stay home from school
- Signs of seriousness or depression in a usually cheerful child
- Expression of a desire to change schools or classrooms
- Sudden loss of confidence in the child
- A new shameful or embarrassed attitude in the child

Any of the signs above indicate that something is amiss with your child. Exactly what it is will come out in the course of the Children's Compassion Remedy.

Children have very little defense against the humiliations of life. They lack the social skills to deal with them. (Not that adults find it easy, either.) A child who has been humiliated needs very tender, gentle handling. If the child is young enough, having him or her sit on your lap or in some way make physical contact with you while you talk is helpful and reassuring. Even older children may allow you to put a hand on their shoulder or have some other physical contact but never push it if they seem uncomfortable about it.

It is extremely important not to try to joke with a humiliated child or make any attempt to make light of the situation. A respectful attitude that allows the child his or her dignity will go a long way toward beginning the healing process. Don't talk baby talk or speak condescendingly to the child. No matter how trivial the event may seem to you, treat it with great respect as the child talks about it. Also, don't discuss the event with others in the child's hearing.

A humiliation is no less devastating to the child than a physical blow and it's wise to keep this in mind as you work together.

Use the Children's Compassion Remedy at the end of this Section to provide help to the child.

Childhood Trauma of Abandonment

There are many things that can cause a child to feel abandoned. They range from the major experience of having parents desert a child to the more minor experience of being left with a babysitter or not taken along on a vacation. Depending on the sensitivity of the child and his or her history, an experience a parent or guardian considers minor can be quite destructive to the child's sense of well being. Because of this, whenever you see a child showing signs of a sense of abandonment, it is best to provide help as soon as possible. What are those signs? The list below may give you some ideas.

- A child who is formerly confident about being alone for appropriate periods becoming fearful

- An independent child beginning to cling to a parent or guardian

- A child who previously slept well beginning to have nightmares about being left alone or related matters

- A child asking for frequent reassurance that his or her parents or guardians will always be available

It is often useful to use the Calming Procedure with the child first before beginning the Compassion Remedy. You will find it at the end of this Section. When the child has begun to relax as a result of the use of that remedy, continue the effort to help with the Children's Compassion Remedy at the end of this Section.

Trauma of Feeling Stupid

There are many children who feel this way in our current educational system: children with learning disabilities; children who are shy; children who do have some developmental disability; children who simply can't speak up easily. Whatever the reason behind the feeling, it is the moments when teachers, fellow students, or parents have said or done something to make a child feel ashamed of that condition that need to be addressed. No child, no matter what his or her IQ or learning ability, should be made to feel stupid! Continual problems in this area cause a massive destruction of self esteem.

If a parent, guardian, or friend was able to provide help every time an incident that caused a child to feel stupid occurred, that loss of self esteem could be reduced or eliminated. It goes without saying, of course, that a parent or guardian must also act to remove a child

> *Example*
>
> *When 12-year-old Ken's father divorced his mother and moved to the other side of the country, Ken felt abandoned. His mother at first tried to talk him out of his feelings by telling him that his father still loved him and he would be able to visit him during the summer.*
>
> *It is almost impossible to talk a child out of such a feeling. When Ken's mother learned how to use the Compassion Remedy, she began to listen to Ken's concerns rather than try to reason with him. As Ken spoke, she gained a greater understanding of some of the ways she and her ex-husband could help their son and Ken became less fearful that he had been abandoned.*
>
> *It takes a combination of compassionate listening and positive actions to fully handle such fears.*

from a situation where this type of incident is chronic. One year with a destructive teacher can destroy an entire education and a child's confidence. When you run the Children's Compassion Remedy at the end of this Section, take note of the names of people who continually appear as causing the feeling of being stupid and when one name reappears with any degree of frequency, take immediate action to remove the child from that influence. Intensive professional counseling is a must for the child who has already suffered such treatment for a period of time. Don't ever underestimate the trauma of such a feeling. It is devastating.

> *Example*
>
> *When Sam's mother used the Children's Compassion Remedy to help her son recover from his feelings of being stupid, she was amazed at the series of events Sam spoke of during the procedure. Almost every one of them featured a neighbor ridiculing Sam for something he had done. Sam's mother had never heard the neighbor speak critically but she had allowed Sam to spend the night on several occasions with the neighbor's son.*
>
> *The remedy helped Sam feel much better. Equally as important, Sam's mother no longer let him visit unattended at the neighbor's house. This helped ensure a similar event would not occur in the future.*

Childhood Trauma of Feeling Left Out

There are many situations that can cause a child to feel left out: cliques at school; a new extended family; the choosing of teams in a physical education class; a move to a new school; etc. Whatever the reason, if you think back to your own childhood, you may remember it as a very traumatic feeling.

If the child seems to need just a bit of help adjusting, the Calming Procedure may give him or her the needed support. If the child's feeling is stronger, be sure to do the Children's Compassion Remedy too. You will find both remedies at the end of this Section. For the child who seems to feel this way chronically, more intensive professional help may be needed.

Childhood Trauma of Betrayal

Does betrayal sound like too strong a word to describe the emotions of a child? It isn't! Children can certainly feel this way and often do. What can cause such a feeling: the squabbling of parents in a messy divorce; the defection of a friend; the telling in public of something voiced in confidence. In short, all the same things that can cause you to feel betrayed can cause that same feeling in a child.

Is it a serious trauma? Yes, because it may set the stage for the child's lifelong attitudes about his or her fellow human beings. Don't ever underestimate its power and do provide all the help you can for a child who is suffering from this feeling. The Children's Compassion Remedy at the end of this Section will help you provide that aid.

Childhood Serious Physical Illness

A child who is suffering from a serious physical illness needs emotional aid every bit as much as he or she needs physical medical help, yet this part of the problem is frequently overlooked. Naturally, the medical handling is of primary importance but that doesn't mean the emotional aspects should not be addressed as soon as the child is well enough to do so.

Physical illness is frightening for most children and it represents the possible loss of everything familiar to the child. It is rare that a serious physical illness does not leave an emotional scar. It doesn't need to be that way. For a chronic life-threatening illness, professional help may be required, but there is a great deal that a parent, guardian, or loved one can do to offer comfort. The Calming Procedure as shown below provides the first help.

Calming Procedure

A sick child of any age can benefit from the actions listed below:

❏ Provide the best quality medical care possible

❏ Create a calm, quiet, predictable environment

❒ Provide extra nutritional support if needed (stress burns more nutrients)

❒ Provide very gentle handling

❒ Give lots of physical contact: hugs, caresses, etc.

❒ Provide lots of softly spoken reassurances

❒ Provide the constant presence of a compassionate adult until the worst of the illness has passed

❒ Give plenty of love!!!

When the Calming Procedure has been done, the child may be able to move on to the Children's Compassion Remedy. Remember the following while you do the Compassion Remedy shown at the end of this Section. Although the illness itself is a traumatic event, it has been found that an illness is sometimes preceded by another traumatic event that lowers the child's resistance to the illness. In doing the Remedy, handle the illness per the instructions at the end of this Section and then check to see if there is a trauma of another sort preceding it. If so, handle that incident in the same manner.

Example

Kathy had leukemia and her mother, Carol, was concerned that, while she was responding to the treatment, her quality of life seemed so poor. Kathy was frightened every time she had to go to the hospital and sobbed each time she learned another trip to the doctor's office was needed.

When Carol used the Children's Compassion Remedy to encourage Kathy to talk about her feelings about her treatment, it was a long process because there had been so many trips to the doctors and hospital.

The time spent on it was worthwhile however when Kathy became less fearful and was better able to deal with the frequent trips.

Childhood Trauma of an Operation

The need for emotional first aid exists both before and after an operation. Therefore, there are procedures in this section to be done at both times. Operations are frightening events for adults who are able to understand the reasons behind them. Imagine what it is like for a child who often doesn't understand. Many hospitals today provide support for children who will be undergoing medical treatment. Be sure to take advantage of such support and supplement it with the procedures below if needed. Unfortunately, there are still some medical centers that do not offer such help. If your child will be treated in such a place, it is vital to offer that help yourself or to arrange for a professional to do so. Without such support, the operation can cause lasting emotional damage to the child. With an emergency operation, of course, such help may not be possible.

An operation is often being done because of a pre-existing health problem and there will be time before it occurs to offer help. Occasionally, it results from an accident and there is no time beforehand to prepare the child. When the operation results from a long-standing illness, use the preceding section on serious illness to address the concerns of the child regarding the illness first. Then address the operation with these materials. Likewise, when the operation results from an accident, use the materials in the section on accidents to address the accident and then use the materials in this section to address the operation.

On occasion, the work done on the illness or accident will extend to include the operation. In those cases, it won't be necessary to address the operation separately. Be certain to check carefully with the child for an interest in talking about the operation if there is any doubt in your mind about whether there is a need. Interest is always the best indicator that it will be fruitful to use the Children's Compassion Remedy to provide emotional first aid.

Preceding the Operation

> **Example**
>
> *When four-year-old Jennifer needed an operation to repair a birth defect, she was understandably very frightened.*
>
> *In the course of using the Children's Compassion Remedy to prepare her for the operation, her mother, Stephanie, realized that Jennifer had a big misunderstanding that was contributing to her fear. Stephanie loved to work on her Singer sewing machine making clothing for her children. When Jennifer had learned she would need stitches to close the surgical wound, she was mentally picturing a giant sewing machine closing her incision.*
>
> *With a child, it is difficult to know what may be most frightening unless you ask. With the misunderstanding cleared up, Jennifer's fears diminished and she did well in the surgery.*

If there is time before the operation occurs and no preparatory help is offered by the medical center where the operation will be done, encourage the child to talk to you at great length about any concerns he or she may have regarding what will be done. Write down specific technical or medical questions and make a point of getting those questions answered for the child by the doctor or nurses providing the medical care. For non-technical questions or communication about fears or misunderstandings, try to answer the questions truthfully and in as comforting a manner as possible. If the child has had prior operations and the fears result from those experiences, it is a good idea to do Children's Compassion Remedy on the earlier operation to relieve the fears before the new operation is done. Remember that children do not require that you tell them everything will be wonderful, especially when you know there will be pain involved. Children can be very sensitive to a lack of truthfulness. They need the chance to talk about fears with a compassionate person who won't belittle them for being afraid or make less of their fears. It doesn't require magic words of wisdom on your part. What is needed is your ability to listen; not your ability to talk.

After the Operation

In addition to the Compassion Remedy which is designed to allow the child to express fears and concerns fully, a child who has undergone an operation needs certain physical and emotional reassurance. The Calming Procedure should be done first to ensure that the child is as comfortable as possible. It can be started immediately following the operation. Then, as soon as the child is able to speak comfortably and has recovered enough strength to talk for at least an hour without excessive fatigue, the Children's Compassion Remedy can be done. Both are given at the end of this Section.

Trauma of a Serious Accident

In addition to the obvious stress caused by the pain of an accident, one of the most difficult features may be the shock of finding out just how vulnerable the human body is. Children often view themselves as invulnerable. If you have a teenager, you probably know how lacking in caution they can be. Even though it is hard to have a child who thinks he or she is invulnerable, it is even harder to see the fear that results when the child loses that sense of invulnerability.

In the course of using the Children's Compassion Remedy to help a child recover from the emotional effects of the accident, watch carefully for the part of the event related to a feeling of vulnerability. While children do need to learn at some point in their lives that the body can be harmed if they don't exercise caution in dangerous circumstances, it is best to have the knowledge survive without the fear that often accompanies it. Use the Calming Procedure at the end of this Section as soon after the accident as possible. When the child has recovered sufficiently to talk for a period of time, use the Children's Compassion Remedy, also given at the end of this Section, to provide additional help.

Loss of a Body Part or Function

The loss of a body part or a function of the body needs to be mourned as surely as a death does. The emotional first aid provided needs to reflect that understanding and concern. Even a loss that might seem minor to you, such as the tip of a finger, or loss of ability to perform strenuous physical activity, is worthy of being mourned fully. The Children's Compassion Remedy at the end of

Example

When Matthew was hit by a car while riding his bicycle, not only was his body injured badly, but his emotional stability was also strongly affected. After the accident, even after the body had recovered, he was hyper vigilant, always expecting something bad to happen.

When his family's minister used the Children's Compassion Remedy to help him, Matthew focused most strongly on the element of shock in the incident. It had truly never occurred to the 10-year-old Matthew that he might be struck by a car. He had decided during the event that he could not trust his ability to foresee danger and that decision was the source of his hyper vigilance.

When Matthew was able to reconsider that decision, he realized that he could use a little extra caution on his bike to avoid a similar incident in the future but he did not need to maintain the level of vigilance he was currently using.

this Section provides that chance to mourn. In most cases, the loss will have been accompanied by an accident, illness, or operation. Do the procedures in those sections first. But follow them up with the procedure here unless the child has obviously included such mourning for the loss in the earlier procedure.

Childhood Physical/Sexual Abuse

The most serious part of physical or sexual abuse, aside from the injuries to the child's body, is the loss of trust and innocence and the feeling of being overpowered. A sense of personal helplessness and hopelessness often accompanies this overpowering of the will, spirit, and body of the child. Rage and destructiveness toward self and/or others are also part of the effects left by this abuse.

As adults we can easily forget what it is like to be overpowered by someone of much greater size and strength. When that abuser is also a parent or person in a position of trust, the overpowering is physical, mental, and spiritual.

> *Example*
>
> *As all too often happens, Sarah's sexual abuse came from a relative she should have been able to trust. Because the abuse was repeated over a period of several years, Sarah had built up a tremendous amount of anger against not only the abuser but the family members who had not protected her or believed her when she finally spoke of the events.*
>
> *She needed and fortunately received excellent help from a psychologist who was experienced in working with this type of trauma but it was also useful for her loved ones to learn the basics of compassionate communication so that Sarah could express herself at home too.*
>
> *Most important was for her family to learn that she needed to express her anger at times even if that made them very uncomfortable because of their own feelings of guilt. Sarah was eventually able to work through those painful emotions but it took some time to do so.*

In trying to help a child communicate about such abuse, it's important—before you begin—to visualize fully what it would be like to have a person two or three times your size and strength overpower you and force their will upon you. You may then be more able to understand the fear, outrage, and grief that accompany such a trauma.

The child who first begins to speak of this type of abuse may be timid and frightened. As the communication continues and the child gains confidence in you as a safe person to confide in, the more difficult-to-confront emotions begin to come to the surface. It is vital that you do not express or feel the slightest bit of shock, criticism, or upset when the child finally reaches the rage and hatred that lie at the bottom of the incident. The child needs to get these emotions expressed before such emotions will relinquish their grip. Let the child scream or rant and rage till it finally passes. Never quit in the middle of this expression of anger or rage.

It takes a great deal of patience and courage to help in this situation. The patience is necessary to coax the child to begin to speak; the courage is needed to continue when the strong and often destructive emotions begin to spill out. Don't even begin the process unless you are prepared to deal with both.

A child who has suffered abuse certainly needs the actions listed in the Calming Procedure as a first step. If you haven't already read about that procedure in the Introduction, do so now. It is also very likely that professional help will be needed for this type of trauma. If it is at all possible, use the resources in the Appendix to find such help. Even a child who receives professional help needs loved ones who understand what he or she is going through and who can talk to him or her about it. Use the information given above to help you do that.

Loss of Close Family Member

The loss of a close family member carries more trauma for the child than just the fact that he or she will miss the companionship of the loved one who has died. It also creates within the child what is often the first awareness of death and of the child's own mortality. A world that may have appeared to have a certain stability and safeness suddenly becomes unsafe and unstable. In helping a child deal with the loss of a loved one, the helper needs to be aware of and look for these additional aspects to the loss.

When encouraging the child to speak of the death, also encourage talk of how the child now feels about his or her own life, safety, and security. Don't succumb to the temptation to alter the Children's Compassion Remedy and inject sympathy or reassurance. The child will get these things at another time. Sympathy is a poor substitute for effective help. It only reinforces the idea that the child is pitiable, helpless, and victimized.

The effective way to help is to keep the child speaking and to help him or her spot those destructive decisions often made at the time of such a loss. If you do the following procedure thoroughly and well, the child won't need as much sympathy or reassurance.

Example

After her grandmother's death, Ashley seemed to be doing well in most ways. In fact, she appeared not to have been particularly upset. But she did begin having nightmares that she was unable to verbalize well when she awakened.

Because Ashley's grandmother had been a great favorite, her mother decided to engage her in conversation about the loss of her grandmother using the Children's Compassion Remedy technique.

Ashley had recounted several times how she felt about the death before she finally realized her nightmares were related. Ashley was dreaming that no one could hear her, a fear she had felt when she saw her grandmother at the funeral and wondered if her grandmother was able to hear her or not.

The nightmares ended when Ashley was able to speak about this fear with her mother.

We have been trained by society to offer sympathy to those who are grieving. It's time to start offering more. What the grieving person—child or adult—needs is a compassionate listener who will help him or her talk at length about the loss; a listener who won't make him or her wrong for feeling angry or frightened by the loss; a listener who will steer the mourner to look at those emotions and decisions experienced at the time of the loss that will have such a tremendous effect on his or her own life.

Loss of a Home

Loss of the family or loved ones who inhabit the family home is covered in other sections of this book. Loss of the home itself is covered here.

Is loss of the actual physical home a trauma? Not always. A simple move from one house to another of equal or greater quality probably won't be traumatic, but a switch from having a home to homelessness or the loss of a long-term beloved home can be.

For the child who has become homeless, the loss of physical shelter is traumatic and will need to be dealt with. A move from a home where a significant portion of the child's life has been lived may also be traumatic. When the loss of a home is part of a bigger loss, like the break-up of the family unit, both losses may need to be addressed.

Some signs that this loss needs to be addressed include the following:

• Grief during the time the move is taking place or afterwards

• Frequent requests to go back to see the former house

• Frequent comments about missing the former home

• Frequent nightmares or bad dreams after a move out of the family home.

The Children's Compassion Remedy at the end of this Section can be very helpful to the child who feels a loss like this one.

Trauma of Feeling like a Disappointment

The feeling of being a disappointment is a crushing blow even to an adult. To a child, it is devastating. No child should have to bear the burden of satisfying the goals of a parent, teacher, or guardian.

The phrase "You're such a disappointment to me" is like a slap in the face and is often used as a battering ram by one person to try to enforce his or her goals and standards on another. No child should ever have to feel he or she is a disappointment.

When a child does feel that way, waste no time in acting to correct the situation. If left unhandled, this feeling will have a very destructive effect on a child's future.

A child who has felt like a disappointment can have several ways of expressing the pain this feeling causes. The way your child chooses is often influenced by the child's natural personality and the number of times this expression of disappointment has been used against the child, as well as the length of time the feeling has been present. Some children express it through sadness and depression; others through rebellion once all hope of pleasing the disappointed person has passed. Regardless of

Example

Although 16-year-old Robert had become quite expert at playing the clarinet, he seemed unable to enjoy the praise he received from others. When his father became very curious about why this was the case, he engaged his son in a conversation on the matter. To his surprise, Robert became quite emotional in speaking of it so the father began the technique known as the Children's Compassion Remedy.

When Robert traced the feeling back to its beginning when he was only eight years old, he realized his grandfather had expressed great disappointment in the fact that Robert had chosen to play the clarinet rather than his grandfather's instrument, the saxophone.

This expression of disappointment took on extra power when Robert's grandfather died soon after making the statement. Robert became better able to enjoy his success once this moment had been viewed

how the reaction is expressed, the help for the child is similar. The Children's Compassion Remedy at the end of this Section will aid you in beginning a discussion with the child about his or her feelings of being a disappointment. The expression of this feeling is often tied to decisions made at the time of the incident.

Trauma of Feeling of Inferiority

A feeling of inferiority is often tied to incidents that are covered in other sections of this book. Helping the child with communication about any losses in his or her life will help with this feeling but it can also be addressed directly with the procedure below.

How can you tell if a child is feeling inferior? It's usually obvious. Below are some examples of ways this feeling is expressed:

- Lack of care about physical appearance or its opposite; obsessive care about appearance

- Timidity or its opposite, a brash boastfulness or need to exaggerate or lie about accomplishments

- An unwillingness to participate in daily activities or accept challenges

- Self-destructiveness

It's very easy to see that the excessively timid child has feelings of inferiority. It's sometimes harder to realize that the child who brags or seems to have a "swelled head" can be suffering from feelings of inferiority as well. A child (or adult) with true confidence and self-esteem will not need to resort to such bragging or self-aggrandizement.

> **Example:**
>
> *Susan felt very inferior to the other children in school. When she answered all the questions correctly on her spelling test, her teacher praised her highly in front of the entire class. Susan's reaction was to immediately begin to worry about next weeks spelling test and whether or not she could do as well. Susan's mother saw the 100% on her spelling test and spoke to her quietly. "I see you must have worked hard to learn to spell all those words correctly," she said. "That will certainly come in handy when you write to Grandma and Grandpa. It's much easier for them to read your letters when all the words are spelled so well."*
>
> *Susan was able to accept this acknowledgment because it focused on the usefulness of her accomplishment.*

Treat any child who exhibits feelings of inferiority very gently. These children are easily hurt by criticism or thoughtlessness. It may take some time for the child to realize that you will not be critical or scornful of him or her. Prior to doing the procedure below, it may be helpful to spend some time watching to see where the child has worked hard and achieved something (even if the achievement is minor). When you spot an achievement, acknowledge it well, not with effusive praise (that only makes a child who feels inferior uncomfortable) but with a quiet comment on how such an achievement may benefit his or her life.

The Children's Compassion Remedy at the end of this Section should help you aid in improving your child's sense of self-esteem.

Trauma of False Accusations

As any adult knows, false accusations can be extremely painful. For children there's an added source of pain since they often lack the skills to be able to disprove such accusations. A false accusation, given enough power by the stature of the accuser, can cause permanent damage to a vulnerable child.

Without the ability to disprove the accusation, a child can be wrongly branded for life—a fact that not only influences how others treat him or her, but also how the child feels about him or herself. As a parent, this is another reason why you should be very careful about making an accusation about your child when you are not certain if the child is guilty.

Certainly when you see a child being falsely accused, it's necessary to take it seriously and do everything possible to make the truth widely known. It's also helpful to allow the child to express fully the grief, outrage, and fear that can result from such accusations.

We've all heard the strength of a child's protest that "It's not fair!" Children have an innate sense of what is or isn't fair and they feel violations of "fairness" very strongly. False accusations strike hard at that sense of fairness.

The Children's Compassion Remedy at the end of this Section is designed to allow you to help the child to recover fully from this particular example of the unfairness of life.

Trauma of Feeling Different

Feeling different can be enjoyable when the difference is one we have chosen, but when that difference is forced upon us by circumstances, we may react quite differently. The loss here is based on a desire most people have to be "normal" or like their peers or people they admire. The part of the situation that is traumatic begins with the first moment the child decides he or she is different and that it is undesirable to be different. The child who never realizes his or her differences or who never sees it as a negative will not need help in this area. The child who is aware of it and dislikes it may need a great deal of help.

In an ideal world, we would all accept and appreciate our own differences and those of our fellow men and there would be no loss attached to it. But this is far from being an ideal world. Children can be extremely cruel to other children who are different.

How can you tell when a child does need help in this area? Look for some of the following signs:

Example

Norma's son, Jacob, suffered from a mild developmental disability caused by oxygen deprivation at birth. He had been teased by other children at school and had reacted by becoming very quiet. His mother was dismayed to see her bubbly friendly baby become a quiet, introverted child.

She sought help for him from another member of the support group she belonged to who had training in Emotional First Aid. Jacob was able to express his feelings about the reactions of other people to his disability after being reassured that he was free to say whatever he wanted without being afraid he would be criticized for his feelings of anger.

A great deal of his outgoing personality returned and his mother made it a practice to see that he was able to communicate on the same subject frequently as he grew older.

- Dressing to hide a physical difference (Example: wearing long sleeves even in the warmest weather to cover a birthmark or scar.)

- Avoiding certain activities because they might show off a physical difference (Example: An overweight child who won't participate in sports but looks wistfully on from the sidelines.)

Ultimately we want our children to have the strength to deal with a difference; not to simply conform at all cost. Making the child feel wrong for caring about a difference is not the answer however. Encouraging the child to communicate fully about his or her feelings of being different is the answer.

Children often make life changing decisions based on such an upset and those changes can be destructive. We need to allow all the emotion to be voiced and the decisions made to be re-examined. By doing this, we help a child learn not to allow his or her life to be destroyed by this difference. The Children's Compassion Remedy at the end of this Section is designed to allow you to help the child to recover from the pain of feeling different.

Jealousy of Sibling/New Baby

It is a very normal reaction for an older child to feel some jealousy of a sibling or new baby. The fact that it is normal doesn't mean we should ignore the pain involved for the child who is experiencing the problem or that we should just hope it goes away. It is possible to help the child get over the pain.

Self-centered behavior is common in small children. In fact, it appears to be behavior built in by Mother Nature to ensure the survival of the child. It guarantees that the child will demand what he or she needs under any circumstances and thus live long enough to gain the ability to fulfill his or her own needs. In most children, the self-centered behavior gradually gives way to a more caring form of behavior as the child grows to adulthood. In some children, the process is short-circuited by traumas or the effects of poor role models.

A child is neither bad nor wrong for feeling jealous. He or she is reacting instinctively. This is important to keep in mind when helping the child. A critical attitude toward the child for being self-centered will eliminate all possibility of being able to help.

Children don't overcome the self-centered behavior of childhood by being shamed or criticized or given disapproval. They overcome it by being able to express their natural feelings to a compassionate listener and by being able to see effective role models who act in a selfless manner. The double value of the Children's Compassion Remedy is that it allows a parent or loved one to offer the child the chance to communicate and to set an example of a compassionate caring adult at the same time.

As the child runs the procedure, he or she may express some strong negative feelings. A desire to do away with the new baby is not uncommon although that may seem shocking to a parent. Don't give in to the feeling or expression of shock. The child will get through those destructive thoughts and make great progress toward becoming more loving toward others if you set the right example and let the child speak freely.

The Children's Compassion Remedy is at the end of this Section of the book.

Example

Five-year-old Shane had very mixed feelings when his younger sister was born. Shane had been the only child for quite a few years and he wasn't sure why his parents felt the need of another child. He showed his anger by pinching his new baby sister when no one was watching.

It's possible that Shane would have grown out of his feelings on his own eventually, but fortunately his aunt was able to speed up the process by engaging him in the Children's Compassion Remedy and helping him open up about his displeasure over his new sister.

Shane's aunt treated him with great respect for his feelings and Shane was able to be honest with her. The pinching stopped immediately and within a very short time, Shane was starting to enjoy the company of a sibling.

The Children's Calming Procedure

Provide the child with as many of the following things as possible.

☐ A calm, quiet, predictable environment. Remove the child from the scene of the trauma if it has just happened and try to find a quiet space where you will be uninterrupted. This will help the child calm down and be more able to speak with you.

☐ Extra nutritional support if needed (stress burns more nutrients)

☐ Very gentle handling

☐ Lots of physical contact: hugs, caresses, etc., as appropriate

☐ Lots of softly spoken reassurances (even a child who doesn't understand all the words will feel the intention behind them)

☐ Constant presence of a compassionate adult until the worst of the trauma has passed

☐ For a toddler, the chance to play act strong emotions using dolls; for an older child, the chance to speak about what has happened

☐ The chance to vocalize rage or fear through crying, shouting, etc., without being told to be quiet

☐ Plenty of love!!!

Above all else, treat the child with absolute dignity. Never tease a child who is upset and never make light of his or her feelings.

The Children's Compassion Remedy

Note: The language used in this remedy is appropriate for most children age eight and up. For a younger child, adapt the phrasing to accommodate the child's language skills. Do not talk down to the child or use baby talk, however. It is important to treat the child in a very dignified way. If you have not already read the Section called Vital Information, do so before you begin this Remedy.

The first step in handling a recent trauma is to let the child talk about it and to listen carefully. Some encouragement may be needed at first. You can encourage a child to say more by use of the following prompts:

1. Tell me what happened.

2. Did anything else happen?

3. Is there anything (or anything else) you want to tell me about that?

At no time during the conversation should you become critical or judgmental. Make a point of always letting the child know that you have heard what he or she is saying. A simple "uh huh" or "ok" is enough to acknowledge that you have heard someone. You encourage the child to communicate fully by avoiding judgmental or critical communication or attitudes and by following the Golden Rules of Emotional First Aid. The child's recounting of the event may run for a few minutes or several hours. Be prepared to listen patiently throughout. If the child has told you about the incident but still has attention on it, ask him or her to tell you about it again one or more times. It may very well be that no more than one or a few re-tellings of the event will prove necessary, after which the child may be feel great relief with no more attention trapped in the area.

Frequently, after telling you about the event, the child feels relieved and has no further interest in the event. If that is the case, end the Compassion Remedy at that point. If that is not the case, ask the child if there is something he or she now feels capable of doing about the event or if he or she now sees some way to handle the effects of the event in a positive manner. Looking at this point of view may help the child feel able to act as cause point in the event rather than feeling victimized by it.

Check with the child also for any decisions he or she might have made at the time of the event. Often a child makes major decisions during a time of loss and it is beneficial to take note of those decisions and to talk about them. Sometimes the decisions were wise ones and the talk reinforces them, but there are other times when the decisions would have proved to be destructive. Once the child has had the chance to talk about the event at length and to begin the healing process, he or she might change his or her mind about the wisdom of such a decision. The spotting of decisions and communication about them with a compassionate listener is one of the most beneficial parts of this procedure. There may be one decision or many. Take plenty of time on this question and give the child the chance to examine all decisions.

If, during the course of doing this procedure, the child starts to speak of an earlier similar trauma, go ahead and focus on that earlier time and ask the same series of questions about that incident.

When all decisions made at that earliest time have been viewed, the child will feel relieved and more extroverted and it is then time to end the procedure.

It can take some time for the process of grieving to come to a closure.

If you feel the reactions of the child to the incident are extreme, use the list of resources in the appendix to arrange for professional help.

Section Three—Trauma in the Mentally Ill

Introduction

Mentally-ill people are best treated by a professional in most cases. Because the altered way of thinking that is part of their illness can be confusing to a layperson, it is much more difficult to provide emotional first aid. However, just as you would still apply physical first aid in an emergency situation to a person with a physical disorder, so you would also apply a limited amount of emotional first aid in an emergency situation in spite of a person's mental illness. The Orientation and Calming Remedies given in the following pages are designed to calm a mentally ill person until professional help can be given.

One of the biggest problems today for the families and loved ones of mentally ill people is the fact that such a person cannot be forced to seek professional help. Unless the situation is life threatening, it is necessary to have the agreement of the person before taking him or her to a mental-health professional. There is a Compassion Remedy given at the end of this Section that can sometimes be used to relieve some of the stress of an emotional crisis. Keep in mind that none of the procedures in this book are designed to treat mental illness. While there is a great deal that can be done by a layperson to help a friend or loved one by using emotional first aid procedures, these procedures will not alter or improve the mental disorder.

The Compassion Remedy is given with the suggestion that it be used only when you are unable to convince the ill person to seek professional help. It will occasionally help improve the emotional upset enough that the person is more willing to then seek professional help. Be very cautious in its use however. While it will not harm the traumatized person if done while following the Emotional First Aid Golden Rules in the Section called Vital Information, it can be very stressful to the layperson who is trying to help.

For mental illnesses that involve delusional thoughts especially, it can be difficult to know whether a trauma is real or the result of disordered thinking.

On the pages that follow, there are suggestions for applying emotional first aid to people with a variety of mental illnesses.

Borderline Personality Disorder

According to the National Institute of Mental Health, there is a great deal more that is not known about Borderline Personality Disorder than is known. We know that it always involves a serious disturbance in how the person sees himself or herself and in how he or she gets along with others. The condition can range from a slight problem that the person is able to control most of the time to a serious problem that is often completely out of control. When a person with this condition experiences an emotional trauma, there is no question about the fact that professional help is necessary.

How do you know if your friend or loved one has borderline personality disorder? Here are some of the signs experts look for in making that determination.

- problems with substance abuse
- sexual misbehavior
- out-of-control spending
- shoplifting
- binging or other food-related disorders
- reckless driving
- mood shifts
- anger that is frequently out of control
- thoughts of suicide and self-destruction
- mental confusion
- boredom
- worry about abandonment

There are actions you can take when the person is having an acute problem or to try to ward off acute problems. The Calming Procedure that follows is designed to reduce the stimulation in the person's environment—a necessary step to help him or her regain control. It is useful to use when around a person with Borderline Personality Disorder who is upset or traumatized. In the event of an emotional trauma, it is especially helpful while you are arranging to get professional help for your friend or loved one.

A booklet called **Coping with Mental Illness in the Family** published by the National Alliance for the Mentally Ill (NAMI) is the best resource available for practical help in an emergency. If you have a family member or friend with Borderline Personality Disorder and do not already own this booklet, get a copy without delay. The address for obtaining it is given in the resource listing in the appendix.

The following are the first steps to take to deal with a crisis or emotional upset in a person with Borderline Personality Disorder.

Calming Procedure

1) Immediately reduce the amount of stimulation in the person's environment if at all possible!

If you're at home but there are other people present, take the person to a room where it's quiet or ask others to leave. The excess stimulation caused by the presence of many people can be a key factor in the distress of the person with Borderline Personality Disorder. Allow only an individual the person knows well and is comfortable with to stay. If you are in public, immediately search for a quiet area where you can retreat Even a restroom will do if it reduces the stimulation in the environment. The inside of your car is also an improvement over a crowded or noisy room. Do not try to reason with or handle the immediate upset until you have removed yourself and the person with Borderline Personality Disorder to a quieter location. If the overstimulation is caused by television, loud music, or other distractions, turn them off immediately.

2) Speak quietly, comfortingly, and clearly to the person.

Simple, clear statements help the person understand what is happening and begin the process of calming him or her.

3) Ask the person what is upsetting to him or her.

Do not expect a clearly understandable answer. Confusion is one of the symptoms of the illness and what the person says in answer may make no sense to you at all. Simply acknowledge that you have heard the response and encourage the person to continue speaking until the signs of upset lighten. Do not argue with the person's statements even if they seem patently untrue or ridiculous to you. A person in the midst of a an emotional upset is not thinking clearly and an argument over the validity of his or her thoughts will only prolong the upset. This does not mean you have to agree with delusions—only that you need to indicate you have heard the person's comments and understood what he or she is saying even if you do not understand why he or she is saying it. Compassionate listening is the key to quieting the person enough to allow the emergency to pass. When the person has expressed himself or herself fully and without fear of contradiction or argument, that person will be noticeably calmer.

Realize, however, that even though the person is now calmer, the upset may be a sign that medication needs adjusting or other medical help is warranted and follow up the incident with a call to the attending physician.

On those rare occasions where the above steps do not quiet the person, seek immediate professional help.

Any person, no matter what his or her mental condition, benefits from the attention of a compassionate listener. But the person with a serious mental disorder needs to have a distraction-free environment before he or she can focus enough to gain from that attention.

The booklet **Coping with Mental Illness in the Family** also suggests, as a way of preventing such emergencies in the future, that you work at creating a very predictable environment for the person with Borderline Personality Disorder. The predictability gives the person a feeling of control over his or her life that goes a long way toward maintaining stability. This predictability includes limiting the number of visitors at one time, setting and keeping a schedule for meals, bedtimes, and other events, and always communicating in a clear, concise manner.

For additional long-term steps toward eliminating emotional upsets, see the booklet mentioned above as well as the patient's doctor for advice.

When violence is part of the incident that caused the emotional upset, the victim can become violent himself or herself. In such cases, it is certainly best to protect yourself by getting immediate help. Don't try to help a violent person yourself. Instead, get your friend or loved one to a professional for help immediately. Most cases of emotional upset do not involve violence and pose no threat to the person offering help. Professional help is still the ideal answer, but on occasion, the person may be totally unwilling to seek such help. When that happens, the first steps toward recovery may be up to those who care most about the victim, his or her friends and family. The Compassion Remedy at the end of this Section will be of help to the victim of Borderline Personality Disorder if you are scrupulous in applying the Golden Rules of Emotional First Aid as you do the procedure. When it is completed, you may find the person is now more willing to seek professional help.

Depressive Disorder

According to the National Institute of Mental Health, the following signs may indicate that a friend or loved one is suffering from Depressive Disorder.

- extreme depression
- poor concentration
- poor memory
- difficulty making decisions
- sleep/eating problems
- loss of interest in things like sex as well as in life in general
- thoughts of death and suicide

The chronic illness of depression can be treated with medication and there is no question about the necessity of having a person who suffers from depression under the close care of a doctor. When an emotional crisis happens, it is also best to take the person immediately to his or her physician.

A booklet called Coping with Mental Illness in the Family published by the National Alliance for the Mentally Ill (NAMI) is the best resource available for practical help in an emergency. If you have a family member or friend with Depressive Disorder and do not already own this booklet, get a copy without delay. The address for obtaining it is given in the resource listing in the appendix.

This booklet lists the conditions above as among the painful and disorganizing effects of depression on the life of the person who suffers from it. Based on those difficulties, the following are the first steps to take to deal with a crisis or emotional upset.

Calming Procedure

1) Immediately reduce the amount of stimulation in the person's environment!

If you're at home but there are other people present, take the person to a room where it's quiet or ask others to leave. The excess stimulation caused by the presence of many people is a key factor in the distress of the person with any mental illness. Allow only an individual the person knows well and is comfortable with to stay. If you are in public, immediately search for a quiet area where you can retreat Even a restroom will do if it reduces the stimulation in the environment. The inside of your car is also an improvement over a crowded or noisy room. Do not try to reason with or handle the immediate upset until you have removed yourself and the person with Depressive Disorder to a quieter location. If the overstimulation is caused by television, loud music, or other distractions, turn them off immediately.

2) Speak quietly, comfortingly, and clearly to the person.

Simple, clear statements help the person understand what is happening and begin the process of calming him or her.

3) Ask the person what is upsetting to him or her.

Do not expect a clearly understandable answer. Confusion is one of the reactions to an emotional trauma and what the person says in answer may make no sense to you at all. Simply acknowledge that you have heard the response and encourage the person to continue speaking until the signs of upset lighten. Do not argue with the person's statements even if they seem patently untrue or ridiculous to you. This does not mean you have to agree with delusions—only that you need to indicate you have heard the person's comments and understood what he or she is saying even if you do not understand why he or she is saying it. Compassionate listening is the key to quieting the person enough to allow the emergency to pass. When the person has expressed himself or herself fully and without fear of contradiction or argument, that person will be noticeably calmer.

Realize, however, that even though the person is now calmer, the upset may be a sign that medication needs adjusting or other medical help is warranted and follow up the incident with a call to the attending physician.

On those rare occasions where the above steps do not quiet the person, seek immediate professional help.

Any person, no matter what his or her mental condition, benefits from the attention of a compassionate listener. But the person with a serious mental disorder needs to have a distraction-free environment before he or she can focus enough to gain from that attention.

The booklet Coping with Mental Illness in the Family also suggests, as a way of preventing such emergencies in the future, that you work at creating a very predictable environment for the mentally ill person. The predictability gives the person a feeling of control over his or her life that goes a long way toward maintaining stability. This predictability includes limiting the number of visitors at one time, setting and keeping a schedule for meals, bedtimes, and other events, and always communicating in a clear, concise manner.

For additional long-term steps toward eliminating emotional upsets, see the booklet mentioned above as well as the patient's doctor for advice.

When your loved one is unwilling to go to a professional for therapy after a traumatic event, and when that person has been stabilized on his or her medication with all physical first aid given as needed, it is possible for you to use the Compassion Remedy that is given at the end of this Section. Follow the Golden Rules of Emotional First Aid scrupulously in such a case, however.

Section Three—Trauma in the Mentally Ill

Manic–Depressive Disorder

According to the National Institute of Mental Health, the following signs may indicate that a friend or loved one is suffering from Manic-Depressive Disorder.

- Extreme depression alternating cyclically with manic behavior
- Serious errors of judgment, especially in financial, legal, and relationship matters
- Disorganized thinking
- Poor memory
- Difficulty making decisions
- Sleep/eating problems
- Inappropriate sexual behavior
- Alcoholism and suicide are common

The chronic illness of manic-depression can be treated with medication and there is no question about the necessity of having a person who suffers from this condition under the close care of a doctor. When an emotional crisis trauma happens, it is also best to take the person immediately to his or her physician.

A booklet called Coping with Mental Illness in the Family published by the National Alliance for the Mentally Ill (NAMI) is the best resource available for practical help in an emergency. If you have a family member or friend with Manic-Depressive Disorder and do not already own this booklet, we suggest you get a copy without delay. The address for obtaining it is given in the resource listing in the appendix.

This booklet lists the conditions above as being among the painful and disorganizing effects of manic-depression on the life of the person who suffers from it. Based on those difficulties, the following are the first steps to take to deal with a crisis or emotional upset.

Calming Procedure

1) Immediately reduce the amount of stimulation in the person's environment!

If you're at home but there are other people present, take the person to a room where it's quiet or ask others to leave. The excess stimulation caused by the presence of many people is a key factor in the distress of the person with any mental illness. Allow only an individual the person knows well and is comfortable with to stay. If you are in public, immediately search for a quiet area where you can retreat Even a restroom will do if it reduces the stimulation in the environment. The inside of your car is also an improvement over a crowded or noisy room. Do not try to reason with or handle the immediate upset until you have removed yourself and the person with Manic-Depressive Disorder to a quieter location. If the overstimulation is caused by television, loud music, or other distractions, turn them off immediately.

2) Speak quietly, comfortingly, and clearly to the person.

Simple, clear statements help the person understand what is happening and begin the process of calming him or her.

3) Ask the person what is upsetting to him or her.

Do not expect a clearly understandable answer. Confusion is one of the reactions to an emotional trauma and what the person says in answer may make no sense to you at all. Simply acknowledge that you have heard the response and encourage the person to continue speaking until the signs of upset lighten. Do not argue with the person's statements even if they seem patently untrue or ridiculous to you. This does not mean you have to agree with delusions—only that you need to indicate you have heard the person's comments and understood what he or she is saying even if you do not understand why he or she is saying it. Compassionate listening is the key to quieting the person enough to allow the emergency to pass. When the person has expressed himself or herself fully and without fear of contradiction or argument, that person will be noticeably calmer.

Realize, however, that even though the person is now calmer, the upset may be a sign that medication needs adjusting or other medical help is warranted and follow up the incident with a call to the attending physician.

On those rare occasions where the above steps do not quiet the person, seek immediate professional help.

Any person, no matter what his/her mental condition, benefits from the attention of a compassionate listener. But the person with a serious mental disorder needs to have a distraction-free environment before he or she can focus enough to gain from that attention.

The booklet Coping with Mental Illness in the Family also suggests, as a way of preventing such emergencies in the future, that you work at creating a very predictable environment for the mentally ill person. The predictability gives the person a feeling of control over his or her life that goes a long way toward maintaining stability. This predictability includes limiting the number of visitors at one time, setting and keeping a schedule for meals, bedtimes, and other events, and always communicating in a clear, concise manner.

For additional long-term steps toward eliminating emotional upsets, see the booklet mentioned above as well as the patient's doctor for advice.

If your loved one is unwilling to go to a professional for therapy after a traumatic event, and when that person has been stabilized on his or her medication with all physical first aid given as needed, it is possible for you to use the Compassion Remedy found at the end of this Section. Follow the Golden Rules of Emotional First Aid scrupulously in such a case, however.

Post Traumatic Stress Disorder

Most people think of Post Traumatic Stress Disorder (PTSD) in connection with war veterans, particularly Vietnam vets, but it can occur in situations far more common than a war. Any form of violence, riot-conditions, incarceration, or other trauma can lead to PTSD.

Example:

After the 1994 earthquakes in Los Angeles, many residents showed signs of PTSD. Those signs included the following:

- Difficulty sleeping
- Loss of interest in life
- Nightmares
- Flashbacks
- Anxiety, agitation, and/or restlessness
- Difficulty with concentration
- Cognitive/memory impairment

Each aftershock of the quake increased these symptoms and added to the trauma. It took the work of many skilled trauma counselors to restore peace of mind to these victims. Unfortunately, the magnitude of the disaster and the shortage of trained crisis counselors meant that many people did not receive the help they needed.

The first action in helping someone with PTSD when he or she is having a flashback is the following:

Example:

George was arrested for a crime he had not committed. Before his innocence was acknowledged, he went through the trauma of arrest, incarceration, humiliation, and financial devastation. When finally cleared, he displayed all the signs of PTSD. His reactions were quite similar to those of hostages in a war as, from his point of view, he had been held hostage for no reason. It took the opportunity to communicate fully about his feelings of fear, humiliation, grief, and—above all—anger before he began to return to normal.

Calming Procedure

1) Immediately reduce the amount of stimulation in the person's environment!

If you're at home but there are other people present, take the person to a room where it's quiet or ask others to leave. The excess stimulation caused by the presence of many people can be a key factor in the distress of the person with PTSD. Allow only an individual the person knows well and is comfortable with to stay. If you are in public, immediately search for a quiet area where you can retreat. Even a restroom will do if it reduces the stimulation in the environment. The inside of your car is also an improvement over a crowded or noisy room. Do not try to reason with or handle the immediate upset until you have removed yourself and the person with PTSD to a quieter location. If the overstimulation is caused by television, loud music, or other distractions, turn them off immediately.

2) Speak quietly, comfortingly, and clearly to the person.

Simple, clear statements help the person understand what is happening and begin the process of calming him or her.

3) Ask the person what is upsetting to him or her.

Do not expect a clearly understandable answer. Confusion is one of the symptoms of the illness and what the person says in answer may make no sense to you at all. Simply acknowledge that you have heard the response and encourage the person to continue speaking until the signs of upset lighten. Do not argue with the person's statements even if they seem patently untrue or ridiculous to you. A person in the midst of a flashback is not thinking clearly and an argument over the validity of his or her thoughts will only prolong the upset. This does not mean you have to agree with delusions—only that you need to indicate you have heard the person's comments and understood what he or she is saying even if you do not understand why he or she is saying it. Compassionate listening is the key to quieting the person enough to allow the emergency to pass. When the person has expressed him or herself fully and without fear of contradiction or argument, that person will be noticeably calmer.

Realize, however, that even though the person is now calmer, the upset may be a sign that medication needs adjusting or other medical help is warranted and follow up the incident with a call to the attending physician.

On those rare occasions where the above steps do not quiet the person, seek immediate professional help.

Any person, no matter what his/her mental condition, benefits from the attention of a compassionate listener. But the person with a serious mental disorder needs to have a distraction-free environment before he or she can focus enough to gain from that attention.

The booklet Coping with Mental Illness in the Family also suggests, as a way of preventing such emergencies in the future, that you work at creating a very predictable environment for the person with PTSD. The predictability gives the person a feeling of control over his/her life that goes a long way toward maintaining stability. This predictability includes limiting the number of visitors at one time, setting and keeping a schedule for meals, bedtimes, and other events, and always communicating in a clear, concise manner.

For additional long-term steps toward eliminating emotional upsets, see the booklet mentioned above as well as the patient's doctor for advice.

When violence is part of the incident that caused the PTSD, the victim can become violent him or herself when having a flashback. In such cases, it is certainly best to protect yourself by getting immediate help. Don't try to help a violent person yourself. Instead, get your friend or loved one to a professional for help immediately. Many cases of PTSD do not involve violence and pose no threat to the person offering help. Professional help is still the ideal answer, but on occasion, the person will be totally unwilling to seek such help. When that happens, the first steps toward recovery may be up to those who care most about the victim, his/her friends and family. The Compassion Remedy at the end of this Section be of help to the victim of PTSD if you are scrupulous in applying the Golden Rules of Emotional First Aid as you do the procedure. When it is completed, you may find the person is fully handled or that they still need additional help but are now more willing to seek it.

Alzheimer's Disease

Alzheimer's Disease is not a mental illness but it is a mental condition that can make it very difficult for a layperson to help in an emergency. In the early stages of Alzheimer's, simplifying the questions in the Compassion Remedy as one would for use with a child can be helpful. The Calming Procedure which follows and the Orientation Remedy which is designed to help a person who is out of touch with the environment are also useful. Do this Calming Procedure as a first step when working with an Alzheimer's patient and the Orientation Remedy as the second step

Calming Procedure

Provide the person with as many of the following things as possible.

☐ A calm, quiet, predictable environment. Remove the person from the scene of the trauma if it has just happened and try to find a quiet space where you will be uninterrupted. This will help the person calm down and be more able to speak with you.

☐ Extra nutritional support if needed (stress burns more nutrients)

☐ Very gentle handling

☐ Lots of physical contact: hugs, caresses, etc., as appropriate

☐ Lots of softly spoken reassurances (even a person who doesn't understand all the words will feel the intention behind them)

☐ Constant presence of a compassionate adult until the worst of the trauma has passed

☐ The chance to vocalize rage or fear through crying, shouting, etc., without being told to be quiet

☐ Plenty of love!!!

Above all else, treat the person with absolute dignity. Never tease a person who is upset and never make light of his or her feelings.

Orientation Remedy

1. Make physical contact with person (hand on shoulder, arm around him/her, as acceptable and appropriate to person).

2. Make eye contact, if possible.

3. Introduce self and ask for person's name. If already known to you, greet person clearly using his/her name

4. Give simple suggestions that he/she can easily and comfortably follow (e.g. "Let's sit down over here. Let's step back out of the way. Let's go in where it's warmer. Let's get you something to eat.") in order to handle any physical needs of person and to help him/her be as comfortable and as safe as possible.

5. Ask the person "What happened here?" or some variation of question as appropriate. As the person tells you about it, use questions to get the incident in sequence if needed ("When did it start? Where were you then? What happened next?"). The object is to help the person get the sequence of events ordered in his/her own mind and to give the person a chance to talk about the incident. Let the person continue to tell you about it until he/she has told the whole story, seems oriented about the sequence of events, and is reasonably calm.

6. Continue with any other actions to make the person as comfortable as possible, offer him or her your companionship, and help the person deal with any needed actions that must be taken. (Calling relatives, making arrangements for care or additional help, etc.)

When the person you are trying to help is in the later stages of Alzheimer's, these two remedies may be the only action you can do to help but they are still a vast improvement over nothing. In the early stages of the disease, as noted earlier in this section, you may also be able to use a simplified version of the Compassion Remedy. You can find the Compassion Remedy at the end of Section Two.

Generalized Anxiety Disorder

According to the National Institute of Mental Health, these are some of the signs you might see in a friend or loved one with an anxiety disorder:

- Never stop worrying about things big and small.

- Have headaches and other aches and pains for no reason.

- Become tense a lot and have trouble relaxing.

- Have trouble keeping the mind on one thing.

- Get crabby or grouchy.

- Have trouble falling asleep or staying asleep.

- Sweat and have hot flashes.

- Sometimes have a lump in the throat or feel the need to throw up when worried.

The fact that the person is generally very anxious should not prevent you from attempting to help him or her when there has been a loss or traumatic event as long as you see that the person also sees his or her physician so that adjustments to any medication can be made if needed and extra help is available.

Once that step has been taken, you should be able to use the procedures in Section One of this book or Section Two for children to provide the needed emotional first aid.

Schizophrenia

According to the National Institute of Mental Health, Schizophrenia is a devastating brain disorder that affects approximately 2.2 million American adults. It interferes with a person's ability to think clearly, to distinguish reality from fantasy, to manage emotions, make decisions, and relate to others.

If you have a friend or loved one with Schizophrenia, you already know how devastating the disorder can be. For a person who has a poorly controlled or severe case of Schizophrenia only the two remedies given here can be used to help.

Orientation Remedy

1. Make physical contact with person (hand on shoulder, arm around him/her, etc. as acceptable and appropriate to person).

2. Make eye contact, if possible.

3. Introduce self and ask for person's name. If already known to you, greet person clearly using his/her name

4. Give simple suggestions that he/she can easily and comfortably follow (e.g. "Let's sit down over here. Let's step back out of the way. Let's go in where it's warmer. Let's get you something to eat.") in order to handle any physical needs of person and to help him/her be as comfortable and as safe as possible.

5. Ask the person "What happened here?" or some variation of question as appropriate. As the person tells you about it, use questions to get the incident in sequence if needed ("When did it start? Where were you then? What happened next?"). The object is to help the person get the sequence of events ordered in his/her own mind and to give the person a chance to talk about the incident. Let the person continue to tell you about it until he/she has told the whole story, seems oriented about the sequence of events, and is reasonably calm. If the person is having delusions, remember that they seem very real to him or her. Do not attempt to reason with the person. Let them express the fears whether you think the event if real or delusional.

6. Continue with any other actions to make the person as comfortable as possible, offer him or her your companionship, and help the person deal with any needed actions that must be taken. (Calling relatives, making arrangements for care or additional help, etc.)

Calming Procedure

Provide the person with as many of the following things as possible.

❐ A calm, quiet, predictable environment. Remove the person from the scene of the trauma if it has just happened and try to find a quiet space where you will be uninterrupted. This will help the person calm down and be more able to speak with you.

❐ Extra nutritional support if needed (stress burns more nutrients)

❐ Very gentle handling

❐ Lots of physical contact: hugs, caresses, etc., as appropriate

❐ Lots of softly spoken reassurances (even a person who doesn't understand all the words will feel the intention behind them)

❐ Constant presence of a compassionate adult until the worst of the trauma has passed

❐ The chance to vocalize rage or fear through crying, shouting, etc., without being told to be quiet

❐ Plenty of love!!!

Above all else, treat the person with absolute dignity. Never tease a person who is upset and never make light of his or her feelings.

In a person with well controlled and medicated Schizophrenia, the Compassion Remedy in Section One may be possible. It may help the person and done per the instructions in the Section titled Vital Information, at least will not hurt anyone. It is stressful for the layperson trying to provide the help however so help given by a professional mental health worker would be preferable in all but the most urgent circumstances.

Obsessive Compulsive Disorder

According to the National Alliance for the Mentally Ill, obsessions are intrusive, irrational thoughts—unwanted ideas or impulses that repeatedly well up in a person's mind and compulsions are repetitive rituals such as hand washing, counting, checking, hoarding, or arranging.

These following signs might help you identify a friend or loved one with obsessive-compulsive disorder:

- Repeatedly checking things, perhaps dozens of times, before feeling secure enough to go to sleep or leave the house
- Fearing they will harm others
- Feeling dirty and contaminated
- Constantly arranging and ordering things
- Excessively concerned with body imperfections
- Feeling ruled by numbers, believing that certain numbers represent good and others represent evil
- Being excessively concerned with sin or blasphemy

When the disorder is not well controlled or medicated, only the following two remedies would be recommended.

Orientation Remedy

1. Make physical contact with person (hand on shoulder, arm around him/her, etc. as acceptable and appropriate to person).

2. Make eye contact, if possible.

3. Introduce self and ask for person's name. If already known to you, greet person clearly using his/her name

4. Give simple suggestions that he/she can easily and comfortably follow (e.g. "Let's sit down over here. Let's step back out of the way. Let's go in where it's warmer. Let's get you something to eat.") in order to handle any physical needs of person and to help him/her be as comfortable and as safe as possible.

5. Ask the person "What happened here?" or some variation of question as appropriate. As the person tells you about it, use questions to get the incident in sequence if needed ("When did it start? Where were you then? What happened next?"). The object is to help the person get the sequence of events ordered in his/her own mind and to give the person a chance to talk about the incident. Let the person continue to tell you about it until he/she has told the whole story, seems oriented about the sequence of events, and is reasonably calm.

6. Continue with any other actions to make the person as comfortable as possible, offer him or her your companionship, and help the person deal with any needed actions that must be taken. (Calling relatives, making arrangements for care or additional help, etc.)

Calming Procedure

Provide the person with as many of the following things as possible.

❏ A calm, quiet, predictable environment. Remove the person from the scene of the trauma if it has just happened and try to find a quiet space where you will be uninterrupted. This will help the person calm down and be more able to speak with you.

❏ Extra nutritional support if needed (stress burns more nutrients)

❏ Very gentle handling

❏ Lots of physical contact: hugs, caresses, etc., as appropriate

❏ Lots of softly spoken reassurances (even a person who doesn't understand all the words will feel the intention behind them)

❏ Constant presence of a compassionate adult until the worst of the trauma has passed

❏ The chance to vocalize rage or fear through crying, shouting, etc., without being told to be quiet

❏ Plenty of love!!!

Above all else, treat the person with absolute dignity. Never tease a person who is upset and never make light of his or her feelings.

In a person with well controlled and medicated Obsessive-Compulsive Disorder, the Compassion Remedy in Section One may be possible. It may help the person and, done per the instructions in the Section titled Vital Information, at least will not hurt him or her. It is stressful for the layperson trying to provide the help however so help given by a professional mental health worker would be preferable in all but the most urgent circumstances.

Other Mental Disorders

The following is a list of mental disorders given on the website of the National Alliance on Mental Illness (NAMI):

- Attention-Deficit/Hyperactivity Disorder
- Bipolar Disorder
- Borderline Personality Disorder
- Dissociative Disorders
- Dual Diagnosis and Integrated Treatment of Mental Illness and Substance Abuse Disorder
- Eating Disorders
- Major Depression
- Obsessive-Compulsive Disorder (OCD)
- Panic Disorder
- Post-Traumatic Stress Disorder
- Schizoaffective Disorder
- Schizophrenia
- Suicide

Some of these have been covered in the preceding parts of this Section. Others are included here although not specifically addressed. NAMI offers excellent information on all of these disorders. If you have a friend or loved one who is mentally ill, NAMI is a great place to start in obtaining information that will be helpful to you.

This book is primarily focused on helping people who are mentally well but are experiencing a major loss or traumatic event of some type. For the person who is mentally ill, the first resource for help must be the mental health professional who is treating your friend or loved one.

People with disorders mentioned here but not covered in other parts of this Section, in a true emergency situation, can benefit from the Orientation Remedy and the Calming Procedure given below.

Orientation Remedy

1. Make physical contact with person (hand on shoulder, arm around him/her, etc., as acceptable and appropriate to person).

2. Make eye contact, if possible.

3. Introduce self and ask for person's name. If already known to you, greet person clearly using his/her name

4. Give simple suggestions that he/she can easily and comfortably follow (e.g. "Let's sit down over here. Let's step back out of the way. Let's go in where it's warmer. Let's get you something to eat.") in order to handle any physical needs of person and to help him/her be as comfortable and as safe as possible.

5. Ask the person "What happened here?", or some variation of question as appropriate. As the person tells you about it, use questions to get the incident in sequence if needed. ("When did it start? Where were you then? What happened next?", etc.) The object is to help the person get the sequence of events ordered in his/her own mind and to give the person a chance to talk about the incident. Let the person continue to tell you about it until he/she has told the whole story, seems oriented about the sequence of events, and is reasonably calm.

6. Continue with any other actions to make the person as comfortable as possible, offer him or her your companionship, and help the person deal with any needed actions that must be taken. (Calling relatives, making arrangements for care or additional help, etc.)

Calming Procedure

Provide the person with as many of the following things as possible.

❏ A calm, quiet, predictable environment. Remove the person from the scene of the trauma if it has just happened and try to find a quiet space where you will be uninterrupted. This will help the person calm down and be more able to speak with you.

❏ Extra nutritional support if needed (stress burns nutrients)

❏ Very gentle handling

❐ Lots of physical contact: hugs, caresses, etc., as appropriate

❐ Lots of softly spoken reassurances (even a person who doesn't understand all the words will feel the intention behind them)

❐ Constant presence of a compassionate adult until the worst of the trauma has passed

❐ The chance to vocalize rage or fear through crying, shouting, etc., without being told to be quiet

❐ Plenty of love!!!

The following Conversation Remedy should be used on a mentally ill person only if it is impossible to get the person professional help. If you do attempt it, review the Section of this book called Vital Information as it is critical that you follow the instructions in that section explicitly.

Compassion Remedy

The first step in handling the emotional trauma is to let the person talk about when he/she first experienced the trauma. Some encouragement may be needed at first. You can encourage a person to say more by use of the following questions:

1. Tell me what happened.

2. Did anything else happen?

3. Is there anything else you want to tell me about that?

At no time during the conversation should you become critical or judgmental and make a point of always letting the person know that you have heard what he or she is saying. A simple "uh huh" or "ok" is enough to acknowledge that you have heard someone. Most people will be very eager to talk to you as long as you remain compassionate and interested. You encourage the person to communicate fully by avoiding judgmental or critical communication or attitudes and by following the Golden Rules of Emotional First Aid. The person's recounting of the event may run for a few minutes or several hours. Be prepared to listen patiently throughout. If the person has told you about the incident but still has attention on it, ask him or her to tell you about it again one or more times.

Frequently, after telling you about the event one or more times, the person feels relieved and has no further interest in the event. If that is the case, end the Compassion Remedy at that point. If that is not the case, ask the person if there is something they now feel they might be able to do about the event or if they now see some way to handle the effects of the event in a positive manner. Looking at this point of view may help the person feel able to act as cause point in the event rather than feeling victimized by it.

Check with the person also for any decisions he/she might have made at the time of the incident. Often someone makes major decisions during a time of stress and it is beneficial to take note of those decisions and to talk about them to a friend or loved one. Sometimes the decisions were wise ones and the talk reinforces them, but there are other times when the decisions would have proved to be destructive. An example might be a person who decides he/she is in constant danger and can never let his/her guard down again. If left unexamined, that decision could prove to be harmful. Once the person has had the chance to talk about the upset at length and to begin the healing process, he/she might change his/her mind about the wisdom of such a decision. The spotting of decisions and communication about them with a compassionate listener is one of the most beneficial parts of this procedure. There may be one decision or many. Take plenty of time on this question and give the person the chance to examine all decisions.

If, during the course of doing this procedure, the person starts to speak of an earlier similar upset, go ahead and focus on that earlier time and ask the same series of questions about that incident.

When all decisions made at that earliest time have been viewed, the person will feel relieved and more extroverted and it is then time to end the procedure.

When your friend or loved one is willing to seek professional help, use the list of resources in the appendix to find it.

Section Four—Trauma and Substance Abuse

A person who is suffering from emotional trauma and who has taken drugs or more than a small amount of alcohol is almost impossible for a layperson to help. In actual fact, such a person is also extremely difficult for a professional to help. If the drug/alcohol abuse is a singular event rather than a chronic one, there is some chance of helping the person after the effects of the substances have worn off. In a chronic user, a complete drying out would be needed before the procedures in this manual would be workable. Someone who is actively and regularly using alcohol/drugs definitely belongs in the hands of a professional. The potential for violence is just too great a risk where there is substance abuse. The Compassion Remedy used in Section One also requires the ability to focus one's attention and to remember the past, two skills that are impaired in a non-sober person.

The only real help you can offer a chronic abuser is to do everything possible to get them into a good rehabilitation program—one designed to deal effectively with the problem.

For people who have abused a substance only on rare occasions, the best help is to use the following Orientation Remedy to handle the immediate danger and then try to get them sobered up. After they are sober and have had some rest, use the remedies from Section One of this book that apply to the type of emotional trauma they have suffered.

Orientation Remedy

1. Make physical contact with person (hand on shoulder, arm around him/her, etc. as acceptable and appropriate to person).

2. Make eye contact, if possible.

3. Introduce self and ask for person's name. If already known to you, greet person clearly using his/her name

4. Give simple suggestions that he/she can easily and comfortably follow (e.g. "Let's sit down over here. Let's step back out of the

way. Let's go in where it's warmer. Let's get you something to eat." etc.) in order to handle any physical needs of person and to help him/her be as comfortable and as safe as possible.

5.   Ask the person "What happened here?" or some variation of question as appropriate. As the person tells you about it, use questions to get the incident in sequence if needed ("When did it start? Where were you then? What happened next?", etc.). The object is to help the person get the sequence of events ordered in his/her own mind and to give the person a chance to talk about the incident. Let the person continue to tell you about it until he/she has told the whole story, seems oriented about the sequence of events, and is reasonably calm.

6.   Continue with any other actions to make the person as comfortable as possible, offer him or her your companionship, and help the person deal with any needed actions that must be taken. (Calling relatives, making arrangements for care or additional help, etc.) Then do what you can to encourage the person to sober up and get help for the substance abuse.

Section Five—Group Trauma

by William C. Foreman, Ph.D., CTC

There are traumatic events that happen to one person or to a small group, as when a family loses a loved one. There are also large-scale traumas, experienced by a whole group of people. Examples of this would include natural disasters like earthquakes or floods; workplace violence like a bank robbery or explosion; and global disasters like wars.

Example:

How many adults in the United States would be able to tell you exactly where they were and what they were doing when they learned that a plane had crashed into the World Trade Center. Research tells us that 80% of adults over the age of forty can give such information instantly and with vivid recall and strong emotion. The impact of that trauma is still present today. Symptoms can range from mild discomfort for those who were only slightly connected to the incident to major distress for those who witnessed it first hand or who felt a strong emotional bond to the victims. Among the most frequently mentioned long-term effects are the following:

- Loss of innocence
- Onset of cynicism, despair, or hopelessness about the future of this country or mankind
- Lack of trust
- Fear
- Desire to withdraw rather than become involved in life

The procedures in this book are designed for use by an individual helping other individuals one at a time. They are effective in dealing with either a personal trauma or a large-scale traumatic event.

When a group trauma has occurred, however, it can be most effective to first use a procedure that can be done with many people at once and then follow it with the procedures in this book done on an individual basis for those who need a more thorough handling than the group procedure can provide.

One group that has pioneered large-scale crisis intervention is the Association of Traumatic Stress Specialists (ATSS). They send a group of Trauma Counselors to the site of a disaster to provide "in the trenches" help for those people most profoundly impacted.

Example:

After the Loma Prieta earthquake in 1989, Oakland, California's Cypress Street viaduct was the scene of a large-scale disaster. The upper portion of the double-deck freeway had collapsed onto the lower portion trapping numerous cars in the wreckage. Rescue workers labored frantically for days to remove survivors and bodies while aftershocks continued to rock the structure. It was a traumatic event not only for the victims and their families, but for the construction workers and other rescue workers who had the grim task of digging through the rubble. While the Red Cross provided aid for victims and their families, the Association of Traumatic Stress Specialists provided a team of Trauma Counselors to help the rescue workers through the trauma that the initial earthquake, the aftershocks, and the rescue work created. After each shift, workers were invited to a large tent right on the site where the "debriefing" took place.

I was part of the team of trauma specialists who participated in that event. Here is a description of the procedures that were used.

The intention of debriefing is to give people some framework for understanding their reactions—and to greatly reduce secondary anxiety caused by the reactions. The discussion should involve issues directly related to the traumatic incident. An educational phase occurs near the beginning of the session with reference to a visual representation of traumatic stress. This provides a framework for the individual's confusion over his or her reactions and establishes common terminology. Coping and communication skills are discussed among the members of the debriefing group. It is pointed out that excess coffee, alcohol, and drugs, as well as survivor guilt and not talking about the experience, can cause the natural reactions to become a life-long disability.

The post-trauma reactions are natural—though not necessarily healthy—responses to trauma, and they can be resolved. Debriefing, along with decompression, helps individuals affected by the trauma regain a sense of control of their lives. Decompression attempts to reframe perceptual distortions and to put the sequence of events into proper perspective, which may reduce future conflicts. It also attempts to bring to the surface issues that, left unaddressed, can lead to the development of survivor guilt.

The intent of post-trauma services is to mitigate the effects of an intensely emotional and stressful incident and, ultimately, prevent chronic Post-Traumatic Stress Disorder (PTSD).

Trauma can transform an individual. Disruption can occur in work efficiency, social life, and family relations. The effects of PTSD can ripple out through significant others and co-workers, whether or not they directly experienced the trauma. Studies have found PTSD symptoms to be diagnosed two and three generations post-trauma.

Certain features of traumatic events are likely to cause PTSD among survivors and rescue workers. The threat of death or serious injury or the witnessing of death or serious injury to another, can be very disturbing and can cause PTSD. The experiences of terror, personal danger, and separation from co-workers have been found to highly correlate with a later finding of PTSD symptoms.

Social and family support have been found to facilitate recovery. Use of alcohol or other substances and avoidance of discussions of the traumatic event have correlated with the continuance of intense symptoms over extended periods.

The physiological reactions during high stress, termed the fight-or-flight-or-freeze mechanisms, can cause distortion of the senses.

Perceptions are distorted and memories seem incomplete or errone-
ous. Immediate reactions frequently include time distortion, tunnel
vision, selective hearing, immobilization, insensitivity to pain, and
dissociative episodes, all of which can lead to blank spots in recall.

Debriefing helps diminish these reactions and their subsequent
distortion of memory. It helps place events during the incident into
proper time frame and sequence. This helps make the traumatic
experiences more real for victims, making them less detached from
the incidents.

When you or a friend or loved one experience a large-scale trauma,
it is possible to arrange for a team of Trauma Counselors from the
ATSS to help the entire group by doing the debriefing and decompression procedures. In the case of a workplace trauma, the employer will find it cost effective to provide such aid since workers who
receive help are able to return to work sooner and are less likely to
suffer stress-related medical conditions. Likewise, municipalities
will also find it effective to provide this aid to their population in
the event of a local disaster. Not all employers or municipalities are
aware that this help exists and it may be up to you or your friend
or loved one to ask them to arrange for such help. The address and
phone number for doing so follows:

Association of Traumatic Stress Specialists
P.O. Box 246, Phillips, ME 04966
800-991-ATSS (2877)
Fax: 207-639-2434

The debriefing and decompression may help those who were not
as heavily impacted by the disaster enough that no further help
is needed. If you, or your friend or loved one, were among those
greatly impacted, the debriefing and decompression can reduce the
level of upset. This makes it easier for you to then apply the procedures in this book to get further improvement and use the resource
lists in the appendix to arrange for additional professional help if
needed.

Simply select the section from this manual that is most appropriate
to the situation ("Death of a Loved One" for example if the person

lost someone close; "Serious Injury" if he/she was injured; "Trauma of Violence" if there was violence involved, etc.) and follow the instructions in that section.

William C. Foreman, Ph.D., CTC, is a counselor, trainer, and researcher in traumatic stress. He is a past president of the International Society for Traumatic Stress Studies and was a member of the International Association of Trauma Counselors. He is also an instructor in Psychology & Criminology, Napa Valley College, 2277 Napa-Vallejo Highway, Napa, CA 94558. Phone 7-1-707-254-8655 Email: cforeman@napanet.net

Appendix

For help if you have a friend or loved one who is mentally ill, these organizations can provide you with great support.

National Alliance for the Mentally Ill (NAMI)

2107 Wilson Blvd., Suite 300, Arlington, VA 22201-3042
www.nami.org Main phone: 703-524-7600 Fax: 703-524-9094
TDD: 703-516-7227 HelpLine: 800-950-NAMI (6264)
Email: info@nami.org

NAMI Utah
450 S 900 E, Suite 160, Salt Lake City, UT 84102-2981
Ph: (801)323-9900 Fax: (801)323-9799
Email: Education@namiut.org Web: www.namiut.org

NAMI Virginia
PO Box 8260, Richmond, VA 23226-0260
Ph1: (804)285-8264 Ph2: (888)486-8264 Fax: (804)285-8464
Email: namivanb@aol.com

NAMI Vermont
132 South Main Street, Waterbury, VT 05676-1519
Ph1: (802)244-1396 Ph2: (800)639-6480 Fax: (802)244-1405
Email: namivt1@adelphia.net Web: www.namivt.org

NAMI Washington
500 108th Ave NE, Suite 800, Bellevue, WA 98004-5580
Ph1: (425)990-6404 Ph2: (800)782-9264
Email: grbopp@charter.net

NAMI Wisconsin Inc.
4233 West Beltline Highway, Madison, WI 53711-3814
Ph1: (608)268-6000 Ph2: (800)236-2988 Fax: (608)268-6004
Email: namiwisc@choiceonemail.com Web: www.namiwisconsin.org

NAMI West Virginia
P.O. Box 2706, Charleston, WV 25330-2706

Ph1: (304)342-0497 Ph2: (800)598-5653 Fax: (304)342-0499
Email: namiwv@aol.com Web: namiwv.org

NAMI Wyoming
133 W 6th Street, Casper, WY 82601-3124
Ph1: (307)234-0440 Ph2: (888)882-4968 Fax: (307)234-0440
Email: nami-wyo@qwest.net
Web: www.nami.org/sites/namiwyoming

National Institute of Mental Health (NIMH)

If you or someone you know is in crisis and needs immediate as-sistance, visit our Crisis page on the web. If you have a general inquiry, use the following contact information to phone or fax us, send us an e-mail message, or write to us.

E-mail address: nimhinfo@nih.gov
Phone numbers: 301-443-4513 (local) 1-866-615-6464 (toll-free)
301-443-8431 (TTY), 1-866-415-8051 (TTY toll-free)
Fax number: 301-443-4279

Mailing address:
National Institute of Mental Health (NIMH)
Public Information and Communications Branch
6001 Executive Boulevard, Room 8184, MSC 9663
Bethesda, MD 20892-9663

For help when a friend or loved one has suffered a trauma, contact the following organizations.

International Society for Trauma Stress Studies (ISTSS)

This organization can provide help when a large-scale disaster has occurred.

60 Revere Drive, Suite 500, Northbrook, IL 60062
Phone: 847/480-9028 Fax: 847/480-9282
E-mail: istss@istss.org

Traumatic Incident Reduction Association (TIRA)

This organization offers training for laypeople or professionals in the use of a technique called Traumatic Incident Reduction. Their website can refer you to practitioners across the country or internationally.

http://www.tir.org/

David Baldwin's Trauma Information Pages

This web site has a collection of some of the best information available on the subject of trauma. Highly recommended for information or links to other organizations that can help.

http://www.trauma-pages.com/disaster.php

Center for the Study of Traumatic Stress

Uniformed Services University of the Health Sciences
Department of Psychiatry
4301 Jones Bridge Road, Bethesda, MD 20814-4799
Telephone: 301-295-2470 Fax: 301-319-6965

United States Department of Health and Human Services

Center for Mental Health Services
See the Services Locator to help locate mental health services in any area at http://www.mentalhealth.samhsa.gov/

P.O. Box 42557, Washington, DC 20015
Call: 1-800-789-2647 Monday through Friday, 8:30 A.M. to 12:00 A.M., EST Telecommunications Device for the Deaf (TDD): 866-889-2647 or 240-747-5475 (International)
Fax: 240-221-4295 International Calls: 1-240-221-4021
Visit the Website: http://www.mentalhealth.samhsa.gov/

Appendix

United States Department of Health and Human Services Center for Disease Control

This website (URL: http://www.bt.cdc.gov/mentalhealth/) has some excellent information on the following:

- Coping With a Traumatic Event: Information for the Public
  How to deal with the stress that can result from a trauma

- Tips for Talking About Disasters
  Resources for Teachers, Children, Adults, Families & Response Workers from SAMHSA, HHS

- The Long-term Impact of a Traumatic Event
  What to expect in your personal, family, work & financial life from SAMHSA, HHS

- Helping Families Deal With the Stress of Relocation After a Disaster PDF (134 KB/9 pages)
  Helping family members deal with relocation stress from ATSDR

- Self Care Tips for Dealing with Stress
  Stress management & how to ease stress from SAMHSA, HHS

- Stress & Drug Abuse in the Aftermath of Hurricane Katrina
  The National Institute on Drug Abuse

- The National Suicide Prevention Lifeline
  The National Suicide Prevention Lifeline is fully staffed to receive all calls at 1-800-273-TALK (8255)

- Suicide Prevention Resource Center
  Includes Hurricane Katrina Information and Resources

- After a Disaster: A Guide for Parents and Teachers
  Information based on brochure developed by Project Heartland

- Managing Anxiety in Times of Crisis
  Resources for Families, Teens, Parents & Teachers

- How Families Can Help Children Cope with Fear/Anxiety
  The Caring for Every Child's Mental Health Campaign

- Children and the News
  General information From the American Academy of Child and Adolescent Psychiatry

- Helping Children Cope with Crisis: A Guide for African American Parents From the National Institute of Child Health & Human Development

- Helping Children and Adolescents Cope with Violence and Disasters. Describes the impact of violence and disasters on children and adolescents, with suggestions for minimizing long-term emotional harm from the National Institute of Mental Health

- Helping Age-specific Interventions at Home for Children in Trauma From Preschool to Adolescence from SAMHSA, HHS

- Helping Teenagers With Stress
  General information From the American Academy of Child and Adolescent Psychiatry

National Center for Child Traumatic Stress

NCCTS — University of California, Los Angeles
11150 W. Olympic Blvd., Suite 650 , Los Angeles, CA 90064
Phone: (310) 235-2633   Fax: (310) 235-2612

National Resource Center for Child Traumatic Stress
Duke University

905 W. Main St., Suite 25-B , Durham, NC 27701
Phone: (919) 682-1552   Fax: (919) 667-9578
Email: National Resource Center

Tips for Finding Help:

Because children and adolescents go through many normal changes as they mature into young adults, it is not always easy to tell whether they are bothered by traumatic stress, grief, or depression. Families can be most helpful if they learn as much as they can about child traumatic stress. Helpful sources of information include the following:

- The National Child Traumatic Stress Network, www.NCTSNet.org
- The New York Child Study Center, www.aboutourkids.org
- The National Center for Children Exposed to Violence at the Yale Child Study Center, www.nccev.org
- The National Center for PTSD, www.ncptsd.org
- The Office for Victims of Crime — US Dept. of Justice, www.ojp.usdoj.gov/ovc
- The International Society for Traumatic Stress Studies, www.istss.org
- National Center for Victims of Crime, www.ncvc.org

There are many routes to finding a qualified mental health professional. Families can do the following:

- Look on the website of the National Child Traumatic Stress Network to see if one of its member centers exists in your city or state. The list of members may be found at http://www.nctsnet.org/nccts/nav.do?pid=abt_ntwk.

- Ask a pediatrician, family physician, school counselor, or clergy member for a referral to a professional with expertise in trauma.

- Talk to close family members and friends for their recommendations, especially if their child or adolescent had a good experience with psychotherapy.

- Contact a community hospital, state or county medical society, state or county psychological association, or the division of child and adolescent psychiatry or department of psychology in any medical school or university.

- Contact agencies in the community that specialize in trauma and/or victimization. These might include sexual assault or rape programs, victims' advocacy agencies, the local crime victims' compensation program, the children's advocacy center, or local domestic violence programs.

Index

Index

Index

Index

Bibliography

Beyond Psychology: An Introduction to Metapsychology, Frank A. Gerbode, Institute for Research in Metapsychology, ISBN: 1-887927-00-X

The Three Pound Universe, Judith Hooper, Tarcher, 1991, ISBN: 0-874776-50-3

Life Skills: Improve the Quality of Your Life with Metapsychology, Marion Volkman, 2005, Loving Healing Press, ISBN 1932690050

Nonviolent Communication: A Language of Compassion, Marshall B. Rosenberg, Puddledancer Press, ISDN: 1 89200-0 6

Beyond Trauma, Conversations on Traumatic Incident Reduction, Victor Volkman, Loving Healing Press, ISBN 1-932690-04-2,

Traumatic Incident Reduction: Research & Results, Victor Volkman, 2005, Loving Healing Press, ISBN 1-932690-11-5

The PTSD Workbook: Simple, Effective Techniques for Overcoming Traumatic Stress Symptoms, ISBN: 1-572242-82-5, Mary Beth Williams, Soili Poijula, New Harbinger Publications

The Near-Birth Experience: A Journey to the Center of Self, Gerald Bongard, Hal Zina Bennett, ISBN: 1-569246-02-5, Marlowe & Company

The Compassionate Life, The Dalai Lama, Wisdom Publications, ISBN: 0-861713-78-8

Your Mind and Body are a Corporation and You are the CEO, Janet Buell, Innovations Press, 2001, ISBN: 1-929830-02- 5

The Body Electric: Electromagnetism and the Foundation of Life, Robert Becker, Harper Paperbacks, 1998, ISBN: 0-688069-71-1

Bibliography

Molecules Of Emotion: The Science Behind Mind-Body Medicine, Candace B. Pert, Scribner, 1999, ISBN: 0-6848-4634-9

Innovations Press

Unique Books
for Visionary People

Innovations Press
P.O. Box 4800, Mission Viejo, CA 92690
http://www.innovationspress.net
lbessa@innovationspress.net

Great New Books, Booklets, and Tapes from Innovations Press

Books

- **_The Emotional First Aid Manual:_** Since CPR was first taught to laypersons in 1967, hundreds of thousands of lives have been saved by the techniques applied by those laypersons. This translates to millions of family members and friends spared the grief of prematurely losing a loved one. CPR—more than any other physical first-aid technique—demonstrates clearly that a layperson using easily learned procedures can save lives and prevent suffering.

  The field of mental health has now made a similar breakthrough. There are techniques in the field of emotional health that are every bit as impressive in their ability to prevent suffering as CPR and they have been compiled in this book, The Emotional First Aid Manual. Now every layperson can learn techniques that will prevent emotional suffering and help restore the happiness of millions.

  ISBN 1-929830-15-7 (paper) $19.95

- **_Burnout! How to Restore Excitement to you Life:_** This unique handbook includes fascinating information on the causes and cures of burnout as it relates to career, relationships, child rearing, creativity, spirituality, and personal improvement. It also has self-help and mutual-help procedures which can be done by the reader to eliminate that burned-out feeling and restore full enthusiasm and vitality to life.

  ISBN 1-929830-12-2 (paper) $19.95

- **_Your Mind and Body are a Corporation and You are the CEO:_** Picture your mind and body as a giant corporation with worker cells making up the body and executive cells making up the mind. Where do you fit in? You're the Chief Executive Officer! How well you understand and execute your role determines how well your corporation functions and how productive it is. This fascinating book lays out a method for assuming responsibility for your own corporation and turning it into a thriving enterprise. It covers the following: how to avoid a hostile takeover; how to improve morale and productivity; how to debug an area that isn't doing well; how to be a first-class executive who has earned the respect of his or her employees.

ISBN 1-929830-02-5 (paper) $19.95

- ***Choices in the Hereafter:*** A small child is brought by his parents to a therapist. What's the problem: He's four years old, reads college texts with ease, recognizes relatives who have never before seen him, and speaks of things beyond the scope of a child. This book follows the extraordinary path taken by the therapist in his quest to find out what makes this child exceptional. *Choices in the Hereafter* addresses such questions as the true nature of talent and genius, the path of mankind and evolution, and the choices that might await us in the Hereafter. (fiction)

ISBN 1-929830-05-X (Hard Cover) $16.95

- ***The Learning Disabled:*** Learning Disabilities are often hidden and are largely misunderstood by the general population. Because of this, they cause a tremendous loss of self esteem to the people who have them. Children and adults alike are taunted by others for their stupidity when, in fact, the learning disabled often have above average IQs. Compensating for the disability can improve school or job performance, but a method of restoring damaged self confidence is needed too. *The Learning Disabled* satisfies that need.

ISBN 1-929830-01-7 (paper) $19.95

Booklet Series — $8.00 Per Booklet

Each of the booklets in our series contain information and procedures that can be used by the reader to help themselves or others attain the abilities covered in that booklet.

- *Increasing Creativity and the Pleasure it Brings:* In today's world, a person who is trying to be creative has a tough path to follow. First and foremost, there's the desire to be able to be creative on a full-time basis weighed against the need to earn a living. There are a few fortunate souls who manage to combine the two desires easily but for most of us, it's a struggle. It shouldn't have to be that way. This booklet is designed to help you increase creativity and be able to earn a living in a creative way.

- *How to Free Yourself from Manipulation:* There's one overriding need which makes us susceptible to being manipulated. That's our constant search for approval, admiration, and appreciation. This might seem like a strange idea. Haven't we been taught since childhood to try to gain the approval of our parents, teachers, relatives and most of the rest of the people on this planet? If you stop teaching children to seek approval, how will they know what's right. The procedures in this booklet will help you free yourself from manipulation.

- *Curiosity, Compassion, and Persistence:* There are three qualities essential in a person who wants to provide effective emotional help to others. Those qualities are compassion, curiosity or interest in others, and persistence. No matter how much training you've had, if you're lacking in these three qualities, you'll be largely unable to help your fellow man. No matter how little training you've had, if you possess these three qualities, you'll be able to help your fellow man effectively. The procedures in this booklet will help you gain those three qualities.

- *Freedom from Self Sabotage:* Do you ever sabotage yourself? Are you a self-sacrificing person? Can you make gains in every area of life but one? Are you restraining yourself from reaching for what you want? Is your progress a series of three steps forward and two steps back? If you answered yes to any of these questions, this booklet contains special procedures created just for you. They are designed to locate the handle the most destructive intentions.

- ***Increasing Your Compassion for Others and Yourself:*** This booklet will help you handle, once and for all time, one of the biggest obstacles in your pathway toward an unbroken state of integrity and real happiness—your ability to have compassion toward yourself and others. And the procedures in this booklet will make an enjoyable experience out of doing just that.

Great New Books and Booklets from Innovations Press

Books	Quantity	Price
The Emotional First Aid Manual	————	————
ISBN 1-929830-15-7 (paper) $19.95		
Burnout!	————	————
ISBN 1-929830-12-2 (paper) $19.95		
Your Mind and Body are a Corporation and You are the CEO	————	————
ISBN 1-929830-02-5 (paper) $19.95		
Choices in the Hereafter	————	————
ISBN 1-929830-16-5 (paper) $19.95		
The Learning Disabled	————	————
ISBN 1-929830-01-7 (paper) $19.95		

Booklet Series — $8.00 Per Booklet

- Increasing Creativity ———— ————
- How to Free Yourself from Manipulation. ———— ————
- Increasing Your Compassion ———— ————
- Freedom from Self-Sabotage ———— ————
- Curiosity, Compassion & Persistence ———— ————

Subtotal ————————

Add $2.00 postage for each book and $1.00 for each booklet.

Total ————————

Over

Name _____

Address _____

_____

Phone (In case we have a question about your order)

_____

Mail order form to Innovations Press
P.O. Box 4800, Mission Viejo, CA 92690

All orders will be shipped within 72 hours.

Great New Books and Booklets from Innovations Press

Books	Quantity	Price
The Emotional First Aid Manual	————	————
ISBN 1-929830-15-7 (paper) $19.95		
Burnout!	————	————
ISBN 1-929830-12-2 (paper) $19.95		
Your Mind and Body are a Corporation and You are the CEO	————	————
ISBN 1-929830-02-5 (paper) $19.95		
Choices in the Hereafter	————	————
ISBN 1-929830-16-5 (paper) $19.95		
The Learning Disabled	————	————
ISBN 1-929830-01-7 (paper) $19.95		

Booklet Series — $8.00 Per Booklet

	Quantity	Price
• Increasing Creativity	————	————
• How to Free Yourself from Manipulation.	————	————
• Increasing Your Compassion	————	————
• Freedom from Self-Sabotage	————	————
• Curiosity, Compassion & Persistence	————	————

Subtotal ——————————

Add $2.00 postage for each book and
$1.00 for each booklet.

Total ——————————

Over

Name   _____

Address

_____

_____

Phone (In case we have a question about your order)

_____

Mail order form to Innovations Press
P.O. Box 4800, Mission Viejo, CA 92690

All orders will be shipped within 72 hours.

About the Author

Janet Buell is an ordained minister who specializes in pastoral counseling and who received extensive training in trauma counseling techniques from organizations like the Association of Trauma Stress Specialists and the Red Cross. Janet has over 20,000 hours of experience in applying techniques like the ones in this book. She has also spent twenty years as an editor and writer and is the author of six previous books including *Your Mind and Body are a Corporation and You are the CEO* and *Burnout, What you can do to add Excitement to Life*.

Contact Us

We would love to hear from you about your experiences in using the techniques in the book or about your opinions of the materials in the book. We hope to improve the book with each new addition so be sure to give us your feedback so that we can incorporate it into future editions. Send comments by e-mail to the author at jbuell@innovationspress.net or to the editor at lbessa@innovationspress.net.

Comments by mail can be sent to Innovations Press at P.O. Box 4800, Mission Viejo, CA 92690.

Compassion Remedy

Use only when you have read the complete instructions
and know how to follow the **Golden Rules of Emotional First Aid**
shown on the other side of this card.

The first step in handling the emotional trauma is to let the person talk about when he or she first began to realize that the event was about to occur and then continue to the end of the story. Some encouragement may be needed at first. You can encourage a person to say more by use of the following prompts:

1. Tell me what happened.

2. Did anything else happen?

3. Is there anything else you want to tell me about that?

At no time during the conversation should you become critical or judgmental. Make a point of always letting the person know that you have heard what they are saying. A simple "uh huh" or "ok" is enough to acknowledge that you have heard someone. Most people will be very eager to talk to you as long as you remain compassionate and interested. You encourage the person to communicate fully by avoiding judgmental or critical communication or attitudes and by following the Golden Rules of Emotional First Aid. The person's recounting of the event may run for a few minutes or several hours. Be prepared to listen patiently throughout. If the person has told you about the event but still has attention on it, ask him or her to tell you about it again one or more times.

Frequently, after telling you about the event, the person feels relieved and has no further interest in the event. If that is the case, end the Compassion Remedy at that point. If that is not the case, ask the person if there is something he or she now feels can be done about the event or if he or she now sees some way to handle the effects of the event in a positive manner. Looking at this point of view may help the person feel able to act as cause in the event rather than feeling victimized by it.

Check with the person also for any decisions he or she might have made at the time of the event. Often someone makes major decisions during a time of stress and it is beneficial to take note of those decisions and to talk about them to a friend or loved one. Sometimes the decisions were wise ones and the talk reinforces them, but there are other times when the decisions would have proved to be destructive. An example might be a person who decides he or she must become very, very cautious in order to never have the trauma happen again. If left unexamined, that decision could prove to be harmful. Once the person has had the chance to talk about the upset at length and to begin the healing process, he or she might change his or her mind about the wisdom of such a decision. The spotting of decisions and communication about them with a compassionate listener is one of the most beneficial parts of this procedure. There may be one decision or many. Take plenty of time on this question and give the person the chance to examine all decisions.

If, during the course of doing this procedure, the person starts to speak of an earlier similar event, go ahead and focus on that earlier time and ask the same series of questions about that incident.

When all decisions made at that earliest time have been viewed, the person will feel relieved and more extroverted and it is then time to end the procedure.

The Seven Golden Rules of Emotional First Aid

Be Persistent

Ask Simple Questions

Show Great Interest

Do Not Attempt a Diagnosis

Acknowledge Responses

Listen — Don't Talk

Be Compassionate — Not Critical